This book is dedicated to my patients.

THE
VITAL
PLAN

An essential *lifestyle* manual
for protecting your most vital asset.

William C. Rawls, Jr., M.D.

This book is designed to aid motivated individuals in the pursuit of optimal health. It should not be viewed as a substitute for competent medical evaluation and care. It is also not intended for use in self-diagnosis and self-help in regard to treatment of medical conditions. Before considering making significant dietary or lifestyle modifications, consultation with a qualified healthcare provider is recommended, especially if serious medical conditions such as diabetes, high blood pressure or heart disease exist.

This book was originally published as, HEALTH FIRST!, An Essential Manual for Protecting Your Most Vital Asset, in 2009. The information was revised and re-published in the present form under the new title:

VITAL PLAN, Inc.
Copyright 2012
William C. Rawls, Jr. M.D.

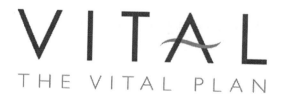

Vital Plan, Inc.
711 Hillsborough St. Suite 230
Raleigh, N. C. 27603

Printed in the United States of America
XXXXXXX

ISBN 978-0-9823225-1-2

LCCN 2009901564

CONTENTS

PURIFY

ACTIVE

CALM

CONCLUSION

VITAL PLAN

Introduction

My first clinical rotation in medical school was on the nephrology (kidney disease) service. Most of the patients were very ill and large quantities of potent drugs were necessary to keep them alive. Quality of life was quite low. It was decidedly not the type of medicine I wanted to pursue as a career. My interest, as a physician, was in keeping patients from getting to that point.

By my fourth year of medical school I had made a decision to pursue a career in obstetrics. Obstetrics dealt with bringing life into the world. It was generally bright and uplifting. The Ob/Gyn specialty fit my personality well. Four years of postgraduate training in obstetrics and gynecology was both challenging and stimulating. Though much of obstetrics deals with healthy individuals, pregnant patients do get sick and helping them get well is an important part of the job. Training in gynecology also included a large cancer service, offering exposure to the full spectrum of medical care. The overall approach, however, was much less drug oriented and much more wellness oriented than other specialties of medicine.

The first ten years in private practice were some of the most exciting in my life. At a young age, I could easily balance long nights on call with a busy practice and at the same time have a normal family life and contribute to my community. By mid-forties, however, worsening insomnia and fatigue, presumed to be related to years of night call, was beginning to erode my health. At first I turned to colleagues practicing conventional medicine for help, but quickly found that all drugs available for insomnia, even the newest ones, were accompanied by significant side effects. For several years I existed in a compromised state, using medications on nights not on call to get enough sleep to last through the nights when I was on call. I finally made the difficult decision to leave obstetrics behind, changing my practice of medicine and my life forever, but not necessarily in a negative way.

Throughout my career I considered health and wellness to be of paramount importance, but as I shifted away from obstetrics and toward primary care, these wellness concepts became the central focus of my practice and my entire life. Thirsty for more knowledge, I dug in my heels to learn everything I could about health restoration and herbal therapy. It was like going back to medical school again, learning completely different approaches to treat the same old problems. I read book after book, studied remedies that have been used for hundreds of years, researched clinical studies, went to conferences, spoke with other professionals well versed in natural therapy. Over time I developed a true appreciation for the difference that the quality of ingredients and therapeutic dosing make in determining a supplement's effectiveness. I attended conferences on holistic and alternative medicine, but retained my ability to apply objective scientific scrutiny. I volunteered at a local free clinic to familiarize myself with the conventional medicine approach to everyday primary care problems, but at the same time searched for better solutions.

All the while, I was working to regain my own health. I began shifting my focus from unsuccessfully searching for a diagnosis to restoring my health. By necessity, my life became very regimented. Moderate exercise, meditation and yoga were daily routines. I became a self-taught expert in nutrition and only allowed healthy foods in my diet. I found supplements that actually helped the sleep problem, without the risk of side effects and dependence. My health and my energy level gradually rebounded.

I had left a large Ob/Gyn practice and started an independent practice based on concepts of wellness. While this transition entailed significant stress in itself, I felt a calling to spread my new-found message. For individuals whose needs were not met by conventional therapy, my new practice would provide an alternative. Motivated individuals who wanted to regain their health, as I had, could find resources to do so. Patients who were not able to tolerate drug therapy could find non-drug alternatives and combinations of nutraceuticals that would work just as well.

Writing a health book was not part of my original intent; it simply evolved while everything else was going on. While brief office visits work in the conventional medical setting, they do not provide enough time to guide major changes in someone's life. I found written information to be an essential part of patient education. Most of the available "canned" health information was not satisfactory, so I started writing it myself.

Initially my writing consisted mainly of short essays about specific topics, to be passed along to patients at office visits. Gradually, the topics came together to explain the concepts of why disease occurs, and more importantly, what to do about it. As it coalesced into book form, I added personal insights and patient experiences to convey sometimes dry information in a pleasing format.

For three years the book existed as a living document, primarily used as a manual for an eight week health improvement course in the office. Maintained as computer text, the book was edited with every question asked and every new concept that came along. With each edit it evolved to be more complete. This final edition, finally ready for print, is truly a definitive resource for achieving optimal wellness and longevity.

This book is designed to provide a practical and comprehensive foundation for health optimization. It was specifically not intended to be a self-diagnosis/self-help book for self-treatment of medical problems—there are plenty of those on the market, some of which are potentially harmful. People turn to self-help books because they are not getting the answers they want at their doctors' offices. Personally, I feel that illness is best treated under the guidance of a qualified healthcare practitioner, but patients need and want more than just prescriptions. It is time for the healthcare profession to evolve beyond this level.

In my office, the health program and the book provide core information for general health improvement. This is complemented by counseling and a set of monographs I wrote called "Health Briefs," which serve to guide the patient in treatment of a specific illness. The entire system is designed to empower the patient to gain control over personal health and overcome disease. Therapy is focused on maximal healing with the lowest possible potential for toxicity.

Of course, I need to note that all patients referenced in the book were fictitious, each a conglomeration of different patients, used to convey ideas. None of the names used here correspond to the names of actual individuals.

The knowledge I have to offer does not consist of miracle cures, as I believe those are few and far between. The miracle is in life itself; all the rest is instinct. Most of us inherently know what is good for us, but we tend to ignore it or lose tract of it. Sometimes we need a beacon to guide us back to what really matters in life. Just writing this book has been a beacon for me. I hope it will be for you.

Your personal starting point, from a health point of view, does not really matter; anyone, at any level should be able to gain benefit. If you have a significant illness, seek the guidance of a qualified healthcare provider, but at the same time, take control of your own health by following the guidelines in this book. If you follow any of the recommendations in this book, you will regain lost health. If you follow most of the recommendations in this book, you will maximize your potential for achieving a fulfilling and healthy life. *I am confident that most health problems can be overcome by improved health habits. Better health is within anyone's grasp!*

The first four chapters of the book are devoted to constructing a model of how and why disease occurs and how it is balanced by the natural healing potential of the body. Understanding these concepts is very important. They are the backbone for making real change. The approach is "holistic" but certainly complementary to any medical therapy you may be receiving.

The remainder of the book is divided into four sections. NOURISH includes five chapters devoted to everything you would ever want to know about food and nourishment. PURIFY discusses toxins and detoxification. ACTIVE focuses on physical fitness. CALM is devoted to synchrony of the mind and body. This concept is useful for developing a practical approach to exercise and stress modification.

There is a lot of information in the book, but it is designed to be a complete resource without reading like an encyclopedia. It does not have to be read from front to back, cover to cover, to be best utilized. Some sections of the book present and discuss concepts, while others stand alone as reliable references on important health topics. Throughout the book there are suggestions for lab tests that correlate with specific topics (noted in by the symbol ◊). These are summarized in an appendix and can be ordered under the direction of your personal healthcare provider. Specific guidelines for what classifies as healthy food can be found in chapter eight. Chapter nine applies the guidelines by teaching concepts of healthy cooking. If stress management is an issue, you may want to turn directly to chapter fourteen. The concepts of the book are extended at with www.vitalplan.com. The website offers additional resources for breaking into a healthier lifestyle!

INTRODUCTION, NEW EDITION

The first edition of this book was born of necessity. Office visits never seem to allow enough time for thorough counseling. Printed information is essential for guiding someone toward better health, but the kind of comprehensive information needed did not exist at the time—so I got busy writing. What started as a collection of handouts coalesced over several years into book form. Though providing information was my primary goal in writing the book, I made every effort to make it easy to read. Dog-eared copies brought in by patients suggest the goal was met.

For this edition, about a third of the information has been revised. I hope that readers find it to be even more user-friendly than the original. One of the biggest changes is a call to dramatically reduce or even eliminate dietary wheat. Mounting evidence strongly supports my observation that most people do better without wheat (white flour and whole grain alike). While this is contrary to the message being sent by the food industry, I would feel irresponsible not sounding the alarm. Taking away someone's wheat, however, is a tough prescription. To compensate, the book offers plenty of palatable alternatives and options for easing into a healthful lifestyle.

A problem with any book is that the information is static. Though the concepts of this new edition are sound, new information will continue to come along. Fortunately, this edition is supported by a website—hence the name change. Through newsletters and information posted on the website, the book can become a living document. Pertinent information can be forwarded to interested parties. New concepts can be explored and new recipes can be added. It is my sincere hope that both the book and the website will empower people to initiate positive, lasting changes in their lives.

Your body is the vehicle of experiencing this life.

How well you take care of your body will greatly influence the quality of that experience.

CHAPTER 1

Health of America

Flying across the country offers a perfect opportunity for people watching. A cross-section of America, young and old, all sizes and shapes, different races and certainly different levels of health, sandwiched within the confines of a jet airliner. For a four hour period today, I will be sharing time and direction with this group of individuals. With any luck, our flight will go well and we will arrive on time at Denver International Airport.

I pass the time studying the people around me. We are all alike, but dissimilar at the same time. The greatest thing we share in common, besides our destination, is a genetic code that is similar enough to define us all as being one species. Beyond this, we are different. This remarkable code allows for such an infinite number of variations that, with the exception of the identical twin girls in row 24, the genetic makeup of each individual on this plane is unique. Different shapes, different sizes, different skin tones, and different hair color. Differences that can sometimes be covered up but not truly changed.

Many of our individual differences can be traced to birth, but many others have been shaped by our environment over time. Choices make us who we are. Choices—possibly even more than our genes—define how healthy we will be throughout our lives. Human nature tends to drive us toward choices that are not always the best for our health. There is a good chance that fewer than half of the individuals around me consume fresh fruits and vegetables with any regularity and a good chance that they survive mostly on a processed form of the corn and wheat harvested from the fields that lie below us. To be candid, most of them are overweight. Of the ones under the age of thirty, most have never had major health problems and, therefore, take their health completely for granted, but a large portion of those over forty have had their lives limited or shaped in some way by changing health.

The flight attendant leans over to pass me a bottle of water, a cup of ice and a package that the airline describes as a "snack." The water tastes like plastic, and I assume it has been sitting out in the sun on the tarmac before being placed inside the plane, but I am thirsty so I drink it anyway. Inside the box there is a small sandwich made with white bread, plastic-looking yellow cheese and what I think may be ham. Also included are a napkin, a plastic knife, fork and spoon set, a package of mayonnaise, a small clump of grapes and a chocolate bar.

I notice the people around me have no problem consuming their snack, but I have learned to be more particular about what goes into my mouth. With the exception of the grapes and chocolate, the other food items do not pass my scrutiny for healthy food and get tossed back into the box. Knowing what to expect from airline food, I came prepared with a fresh green salad, an apple, and some fresh mixed nuts, choices that I think will be better for my health.

The luxury of having time to contemplate our health is a fairly recent phenomenon. One hundred years ago people in America had little opportunity to consider the matter. Consuming healthy food was not nearly as much a concern as simply having something to eat. For much of the population, having enough to eat meant back-breaking labor from dusk till dawn. Life was not easy; risks of trauma, infection and malnutrition were high.

My great grandfather was a horse-and-buggy doctor of that era. Compared to today, essentially no health care system existed in his time.

All of the technology available to him was packed into a small black bag, and the nearest hospital was far, far away. The lack of adequate healthcare meant that people regularly died of diseases that could be easily treated today. Shockingly, 25% of children perished before their first year of life, and infections and accidents claimed the lives of many young adults long before they had an opportunity to develop the chronic diseases that we now commonly associate with aging.

Our present day healthcare system has done a wonderful job of relieving us of many of those past-day maladies, but the question as to whether the overall health potential of the average middle-aged American has been improved is still unanswered. A higher percentage of people are living past middle age, but are they reaching their peak life expectancy *and* their peak health expectancy? Disease is still with us, but it seems to be changing. The diseases more commonly associated with aging seem to be on the rise in younger individuals. Conditions such as diabetes, arthritis, heart disease, and most threatening of all, cancer, are becoming almost ordinary in forty- and even thirty-year-olds.

This surprising bit of reality comes at a time when our country seems to have an acute focus on health. A whopping 15% of our economy is devoted exclusively to health care. Advertisements by pharmaceutical companies now dominate television, and virtually every magazine at the newsstand regularly features articles on health. Longevity and vitality appear to be for sale. Clever displays hawk endless varieties of vitamin drinks, "healthy" snack bars, and processed "health" foods. In terms of money spent, the United States should be the healthiest place on the planet.

Even so, the majority of Americans are far from reaching their maximum health potential. The sad fact of the matter is that even with all the hype over diet and health, more people than ever are either unwilling or unsure of how to take control of their own health. The pressures of modern life tend to perpetuate unhealthy lifestyles. Though healthy food choices are widely available, people regularly eat on the run, choosing foods that are more convenient than nutritious. With most jobs being indoors, physical activity has become optional and the perceived stress of living is at an all-time high. The industrial machine that has made America great has also left us with an unparalleled mix of toxins in the environment.

Instead of focusing on health, diet and lifestyle changes are instead focused on weight loss and the treatment of disease has been left almost exclusively in the hands of pharmaceutical companies. Instead of eradicating disease, modern pharmaceuticals and surgery are allowing people to *live with* disease. Ironically, the overall health potential of the average person today may actually be declining, despite some of the most expensive healthcare in the world.

Modern pharmaceuticals prolong life and decrease symptoms, but rarely restore normal health. The actual incidence of disease, including cancer, is on the rise. Until we begin to address the underlying causes of disease, instead of just treating the symptoms, the incidence of chronic disease will likely continue to rise.

We are each interested in our own personal health. Conventional medicine does offer answers and hope for some people, but there is more to health than just a prescription. All of the healthcare options at our disposal are nothing without the healing potential that lies within each of us. The key to maximizing this healing potential is making good health choices.

The pilot breaks in over the loudspeaker to announce our landing in Denver. Everyone on the plane seems to breathe a collective sigh of relief and individually each person prepares for landing. Finally, at the gate with the seatbelt sign off, we squash ourselves into the aisle in anticipation of the door opening. As we file out, it feels good to stretch, and some of the collective stress from being cooped up in a confined space rolls off my shoulders. Next stop is baggage claim, then on to the rental car agency and out onto the highway.

It is still early afternoon, and the traffic is not too heavy. Denver is a great city, but with the summer smog stacking up against the Rockies, I'm glad to be heading into mountains above it all. Through the haze I can make out the snow-capped peaks near Rocky Mountain National Park in the distance. I look forward to the peace, quiet, rest and relaxation that I know higher elevations will bring. For me, this is a very important health choice.

CHAPTER 2

Health and Disease in the Balance

Hiking is a favorite pastime, and Rocky Mountain National Park is a favorite place. Though I live on the coast, the Rockies offer a perfect place to "get away from it all." The park includes some of the highest mountains in the lower forty-eight. The rugged terrain and thin air challenge my abilities and test my limits. Though the trails do not change from year-to-year, my ability to conquer them certainly has.

The last time I hiked the Rockies was about three years prior, with two teenagers. Even in this short time period, I can tell a difference. My energy level is just not the same. The resilience of my younger years seems to have ebbed, and sleep does not come as easily as it once did. Certainly my condition would not be described as disease or even poor health, but it is not perfect either. I guess you could call it aging, but I'm not quite willing to accept that reality. I commonly see these same symptoms in many patients over age forty. Tiredness and loss of energy are some of the most common complaints I hear. In fact,

I would say most patient's complaints are non-specific and do not amount to enough to be classified as classic textbook disease processes.

In western medicine we typically define a disease process as a collection of symptoms resulting from a derangement of the normal processes of the body. Standard training in medical school typically focuses on evaluating signs and symptoms of disease to arrive at a diagnosis, followed by treatment, usually with drugs or surgery. Goals of achieving optimal long-term health often remain secondary concerns. The seemingly most important part of evaluating disease, discovering the root causes, is most often glossed over. When the focus of therapy is directed predominantly toward relieving the signs and symptoms of disease, discovering root causes becomes somewhat irrelevant.

The western medical approach works best when patients are comfortably classified with a diagnosis. A firm diagnosis allows a specific treatment protocol, much easier for the physician and patient alike. A very large amount of our healthcare resources are devoted to defining a specific diagnosis. Even so, a significant number of patients present with non-specific symptoms that elude the label of an absolute diagnosis, complicating treatment and often leaving the patient frustrated. Over the years of practicing medicine I have been gradually shifting away from this "classify and categorize" approach toward more of a "cause and effect" approach.

Disease does not just fall out of the sky. Understanding the underlying causes of disease is the key to achieving optimal long-term health.

Disease can come on suddenly, as with an infection or accident, but most of the time disease is insidious, with symptoms occurring long before a diagnosis is evident. Looking for causes, even before a diagnosis is made, offers a whole new approach to healing. Interestingly, once you start looking for causes, you will find they are similar for many, if not most, diseases. Looking at disease in this fashion is actually simpler and alleviates the constraints of an absolute diagnosis. Primary therapy to counteract the forces of disease can begin immediately for any situation, even before symptoms begin to occur.

The next chapter is devoted to defining the causes of disease, but for now, we can collectively refer to these combined factors simply as the "forces of disease." We are continually exposed to these forces, and gradual, cumulative damage to the body is inevitable. If it were not for the healing systems of the body always at work repairing any damage that occurs, our day-to-day survival would be somewhat limited. Considering the abuse the human body receives over a lifetime (much of it self-induced), the magnitude of the healing potential of the human body is absolutely astounding.

From the day we take our first breath, a tug of war begins between the forces of disease and the healing systems of the body. This struggle will last a lifetime. If these two forces are held in balance, an equilibrium is reached that can be referred to as "good health." Early in life good health is easy to maintain because little damage has accumulated and the healing systems of the body are in prime working order. Up until age thirty most people can live anyway they want to and still expect to feel good most of the time (Figure 1). Staying out all night, smoking cigarettes, eating fast food and living life on the edge does not impact health significantly at that point.

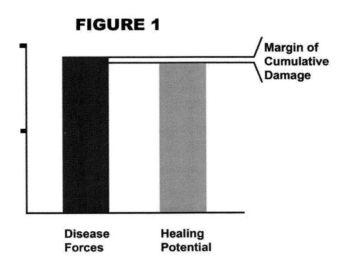

FIGURE 1

Margin of Cumulative Damage

Disease Forces

Healing Potential

The invincibility of youth does not last forever. Without careful attention, damage caused by the forces of disease begins to add up, and the healing capacity of the body becomes compromised and cannot keep pace. As the gap widens between these two forces, the difference can be referred to as "cumulative damage." (Figure 2).

FIGURE 2

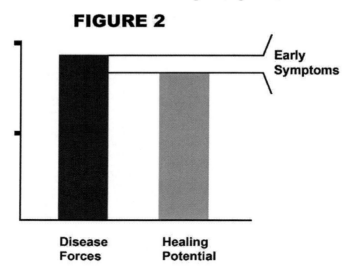

Initially this discrepancy shows up as non-specific symptoms such as fatigue and loss of energy, irritability, weight gain, irregular periods, and other such complaints—because of genetic variation, symptoms may be different for different individuals. As the discrepancy becomes more pronounced, overt disease develops that can be classified, categorized, and located within the pages of a medical textbook (Figure 3).

FIGURE 3

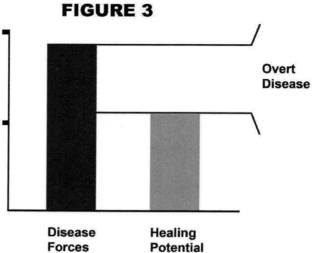

Most of us, by early- to mid-forties, will have some early symptoms of disease and will be modeled by Figure 2. By age fifty, many will be on medications and will look more like Figure 3. The whole situation is a progressive downhill slide, unless you change the way you look at disease. Understanding the underlying causes of disease allows an opportunity to regain the equilibrium of good health by appropriate lifestyle and dietary modifications. By lessening the forces of disease, the healing potential of the body will be given an opportunity to rebound—maybe not to the level of our youth, but enough to restore and maintain good health (Figure 4). **Compromise is in order, but isn't good health worth it?**

FIGURE 4

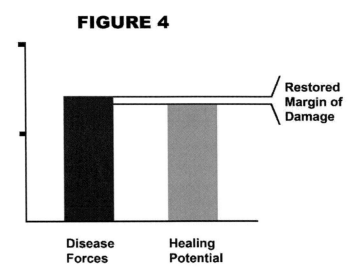

I think about these concepts as I break through the tree line and head across the side of a mountain along a moderately steep, rocky trail. I still have some of my youthful resilience left but would like to have the energy to continue with activities of this sort for many years into the future. I can handle compromise. I have already made some changes in my diet and lifestyle and am willing to make more. Having the health to enjoy life is worth the tradeoff. With maturity and knowledge gained over the years, I can even do some things I would not have been able to accomplish in my youth. With the right compromises I can envision the possibility of my senior years being savored rather than just endured (Figure 5).

FIGURE 5

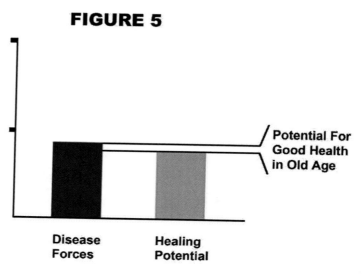

The trail leads to a saddle between two mountaintops. The vastness has the feel of being infinite. Looking out from the saddle to the east I see a small glacier made of leftover snow pack. The base lies at my feet and extends down into a valley between two shear rock faces. In the valley below, elk appear to be so close that I could touch them, yet they are a mile or more away. The air is so clean and dry that the views seem surreal. It is interesting how being part of such a huge expanse can bring one's personal life into focus.

Coming to grips with my own health and wellness has been important on a personal level, but it has also influenced the way I practice medicine. It started with a goal to do more than just pass out prescriptions. Addressing the causes of disease certainly makes more sense than just treating symptoms alone. I was aware that other providers across the country had incorporated alternative therapies and less toxic natural therapies into their practices with very good results, but I also knew that of all the ways that I could help my patients, none was more important than teaching them how to help themselves.

CHAPTER 3

A New Style of Healthcare

Making an effort to understand the causes of disease offers a whole new approach to the treatment of disease. Virtually all diseases can be traced back to common origins. The trick is doing something about them. Offering patients better health choices requiring substantial lifestyle changes, admittedly, is not an easy sell. Changing the way people live is such a difficult task that conventional medicine generally pays little attention to the concept. Treating symptoms is easier. I can tell you from experience that handing a patient drug samples and a prescription with a reassuring pat on the back generally goes over much better than providing good sound advice alone. The act of giving someone some "thing" feels good to the doctor and the patient alike and somehow, by itself, helps to make the situation better.

Unfortunately, the "make the situation better" part is short-lived, as side effects are common and drugs are mainly designed to treat symptoms. **Treating symptoms alone generally does not cure disease.** Symptoms worsen as the forces of disease add cumulative damage to the body, often with more drugs soon to follow. Frequently the drugs become part of the problem. For the early part of my career I practiced in this fashion. I would listen to patients' symptoms, fit them into the diagnostic category matching the proper medical code, and compassionately write out prescriptions to relieve their suffering. Sometimes it actually worked. Often, however, patients would have significant side effects to medications, would stop taking their medications all together, or would just become more ill.

As my practice evolved, I found myself asking patients about what they ate and how much stress affected their lives. I constructed a questionnaire to help me hone in on the contribution of the different factors of disease to a patient's symptom complex. This process often allowed me to bring that person "on board" in the healing process. With proper direction, the patient could take an active role in improving his or her own well-being. For a motivated individual, lifestyle and dietary changes could be, and should be, first-line therapy. Over time, this concept became as important to me as handing out a prescription.

I do understand that alleviating symptoms is an important part of therapy when someone is sick. Symptoms can be not only quite bothersome, but also frightening, and thus a barrier to healing; however, relieving symptoms should not be limited to conventional pharmaceuticals alone. Appropriate combinations of natural supplements can be as effective as drug therapy, usually with lower potential for toxicity. Yoga, meditation therapy, physical therapy, massage therapy, and acupuncture have stood the test of time as valuable healing modalities. Alleviating symptoms, while at the same time helping the patient make better health choices, is an important step toward making the patient well.

As I began to develop a reputation for offering more than just drugs, patients who had not tolerated conventional medications and therapy began to show up on my doorstep searching for other options. Often frustrated and dissatisfied, they tended to be very motivated to try whatever I had to offer. Sarah was one of those patients.

Sarah had been waiting for a diagnosis for over six weeks. She had been to see three different physicians and no one had been able to give her absolute answers. The problem started a little over a year ago when she went to her primary care provider with complaints of acid reflux and anxiety. Prescriptions were given for a medication to stop acid production in her stomach and something to calm her nerves. Both medications worked, and Sarah was able to continue with life; however, her symptoms began to reoccur and other symptoms began to develop.

The burning in her throat was only kept at bay if she took the medication every day. Gas, bloating, and abdominal cramping, which previously had been only minor annoyances, were now becoming a major concern. An evaluation by a gastroenterologist included a CT scan, colonoscopy and other tests. Except for mild esophageal irritation and early signs of an ulcer, all of the studies were negative. She was told to continue the antacid medication and was given an anti-spasm medication. In retrospect, she related that she did feel better after the endoscopies, which had included complete bowel preps, but the respite was short lived.

Her ability to handle day-to-day stress slowly began to deteriorate. Worsening anxiety often left her agitated by the end of the day. Her first panic attack was a real shock. Under the advice of her primary care provider she stepped up taking the anti-anxiety medication to several times each day. She found that she could not sleep at night without it. An anti-hypertensive drug was added to manage rising blood pressure. Routine blood tests discovered a mildly elevated fasting blood sugar, suggesting that she may also be developing adult onset diabetes. With each week she became increasingly fatigued, often to the point that working a full day was nearly impossible.

Most recently Sarah was being seen by a neurologist for symptoms of burning, tingling and numbness in her hands and feet associated with muscle pain and spasm. These symptoms were the most disconcerting of all. In her mind, a disease such as multiple sclerosis was a real concern. She had undergone a battery of tests and was now waiting for results.

By the time Sarah made her way to my office, she was taking six different medications and felt worse than ever. Sitting across from me in the exam room, with elbows on knees and face mashed into her hands, she was a true picture of despair. At age 43 she was not happy with life and was quite sure that she had some terrible illness, yet to be diagnosed. In the past I would have had little to offer but sympathy, but by looking at her situation from a different point of view, I definitely had some positive advice. Often a thorough medical evaluation is necessary, but therapy should not await a diagnosis. Therapy in the form of reducing the causative factors of disease can begin immediately. As the healing potential of the patient recovers, symptoms often improve, even before a final diagnosis is made.

A prerequisite for using this approach is recognizing that chronic diseases involve the whole body. This is not always readily apparent. A condition as seemly simple as a fungal infection of the toe is a red flag that the entire immune system is not functioning properly. Treating only the toe and not addressing widespread immune dysfunction is an open door for other chronic conditions that will inevitably show up.

If you distinguish that chronic disease is a reflection of dysfunction in the body's healing systems, then it should not be a surprise to find so many individuals with more than one chronic disease process. Chronic sinusitis and gastrointestinal problems often go hand-in-hand. Hypertension, arthritis, diabetes and elevated cholesterol rarely show up as isolated conditions, as a majority of patients in primary care waiting rooms across America can attest. This fact alone would suggest that chronic diseases have common origins.

Many individuals, including some health care providers, have the misconception that the origins of most diseases are difficult to define; that disease just happens, and the best way to deal with disease is by treating its symptoms. This is far from being the case, as all things that occur in the natural world have causes, including disease. When I was first exploring this concept, I came upon the last chapter of my 30 year old biochemistry text (the part we never got to) which delineated the known causes of disease. A surprisingly short list of categories was offered. With further reading and research, I have refined the list a bit, but the take away message is fundamental: **all diseases have common roots within a small number of well-defined categories of causes.**

1. **Oxidative stress:** exposure to free radicals generated by metabolic processes and immune system function is the most important factor in aging.

2. **Exposure to toxins:** sources suggest that upwards of 200,000 man-made chemicals have made their way into the environment over the past one hundred years.
3. **Malnutrition:** our food supply, characterized by excessive glucose and abnormal fat, is also profoundly deficient in nutrients and fiber.
4. **Emotional stress:** emotional stress plays a role in most disease processes.
5. **Physical stress:** basic wear and tear, cold and heat.
6. **Microbes:** bacteria, viruses, fungi, and protozoa have been factors of disease since life began.
7. **Radiation:** both ionizing and non-ionizing radiation have adverse effects on tissues of the human body.

Genetics: the deciding factor. Because we all have genes that are unique, exposure to the same sets of risk factors results in different diseases for different individuals.

What a radical concept! It implies that not only do all diseases have common causes but they also have common roots in prevention and treatment. This profound bit of insight certainly begs the question: why does modern medicine seem to be ignoring this important information? The answer lies in human nature itself. Treating disease by removing the causes requires effort, whereas taking a pill is a much easier way to control symptoms. Also, the causes of disease are very much a part of life itself and eliminating them would be impossible. Lessening their impact, however, *is* an option—one to which more of us should be paying attention. Understanding these causative factors offers a unique opportunity to alter our destiny. We can, in essence, cut disease off at the pass just by making intelligent choices in the way we conduct our lives.

Before I could help Sarah with changes that she was going to have to make to alter her own destiny, I needed her to understand these basic concepts. Even when an absolute diagnosis seems elusive, identifying causative factors can open an avenue toward healing. Knowing everything there is to know about the causes of disease is not necessary, but a basic understanding of these factors does answer many questions that patients have about illness. Gaining this type of knowledge offers the patient control and alleviates fear. This, in itself, is a positive healing force.

Understanding basic information about the causes of disease is an absolute necessity for understanding health. Just as it would be unwise to enter a battle without obtaining intelligence information about the enemy, it would be unwise to try to improve your health without knowing about the forces working in opposition to that goal.

THE SEVEN BASIC CAUSES OF DISEASE

Any discussion about the causes of disease must start with a living cell. There are thousands of different types of cells in the human body, but they all share some common features. A living cell can be thought of three-dimensionally as a blob of gel surrounded by a thin membrane holding it all together. Suspended in the middle, almost like an egg yolk, is the nucleus. The nucleus contains chromosomes that hold DNA, the blueprint for all vital functions of the cell. Also suspended within the gel that we call "cytoplasm" are the functional parts of the cell. **All functions of the cell require energy; yet, paradoxically, this basic necessity of life is the root of one of the main causes of aging and disease.**

1 | OXIDATIVE STRESS

Oxidative stress, a term unfamiliar to most people, is possibly the most significant overall factor in aging. The most ubiquitous factor of disease, oxidative stress, is continuously present in all living things and is definitely one to know something about. Cancer, atherosclerosis, arthritis, and inflammatory conditions all have direct links to oxidative stress; in fact, most disease processes have some link to oxidative stress. What is this peculiar-sounding term? The answer is right under your nose.

Take in a deep breath. About 20% of the air you just inhaled is composed of oxygen. Oxygen, a necessity of life that we sometimes take for granted, is actually a potently toxic substance. It is so toxic, in fact, that it took life on earth a couple of billion years to figure out how to use it in energy production.

All living things derive energy by breaking down molecules containing hydrogen and carbon. Fat and sugar are examples of hydrocarbon molecules. When the chemical bonds of hydrocarbon molecules are broken, a small amount of energy is released. Production of energy from this basic chemical reaction was enough to get life started here on earth, but only allowed a marginal foothold. More energy was a necessity for life to truly thrive—oxygen was the key ingredient. Throwing oxygen into the mix was like throwing gasoline onto a fire; an organism could produce ten times the amount of energy from the same amount of hydrocarbon. This little metabolic trick turned out to be the real key to the success of life on earth...but it came with a price.

In high school science class you learned that plants use energy from the sun to make glucose and animal cells, in turn, can use glucose as a primary energy source or can turn it into fat for storage of energy. The basic chemical reaction of combining glucose or fat with oxygen to release energy with the end products of water and carbon dioxide completes one of the most important cycles of life.

$$C_6H_{12}O_6 \text{ (glucose)} + O_2 \rightarrow CO_2 + H_2O + \text{ENERGY!}$$

For this seemly simple reaction to occur, the oxygen molecule must break apart into two very reactive components. These reactive components are "electron greedy" and pluck electrons off of molecules such as glucose. When exposed to these reactive components, the glucose molecule becomes unstable, and the chemical bonds are easily broken, thus releasing energy.

The reactive oxygen components belong to a wider group of chemical substances generically referred to as "free radicals." Free radicals occur in most kinds of chemical reactions and, of course, there are many chemical reactions occurring in the human body at any given second. The fact that free radicals propel a chemical reaction in a forward direction is necessary for life to occur, but with any given reaction, there is always collateral damage. These reactive chemical substances steal electrons from other adjacent molecules, thus damaging and weakening vital components of a living cell.

The process of free radicals "stealing" electrons from other molecules is called oxidation, and it occurs in nature almost continuously. Rust is an example of oxidation. To visualize the process of oxidation in action, cut an apple in half and leave it on the counter. Oxidation is represented by the brown color that rapidly forms when the cut surface is exposed to oxygen in the air. The peel would normally protect the apple from oxidation.

Take another apple, cut it in half, and rub lime juice all over the cut surface. Notice the apple does not turn brown as rapidly. The vitamin C in the lime acts as an antioxidant that protects the tissue from oxidation. Vitamin C and a host of other antioxidants protect us internally from oxidation. We could not survive without antioxidants.

Within living cells, energy production is confined to small, oval-shaped structures called "mitochondria" that are strategically distributed throughout the cytoplasm. Think of them as microscopic power plants, constantly churning out raw energy. Free radicals are an obligatory byproduct of this intense energy production. Not being completely contained within the mitochondria, free radicals shoot off like sparks in every direction. Like microscopic firecrackers going off inside the cell, they have the propensity to damage all structures, including cell membranes, proteins that compose the functional parts of the cell, and very importantly, our DNA. No structures, however, take more of the brunt of the damage than the mitochondria themselves. **A gradual decline in energy production by damaged mitochondria is one reason we slow down as we age.**

Though all cells of the body are exposed to the damaging effects of free radicals, some carry more of a burden than others. The cells of metabolically active tissues require more energy and, therefore, have a higher propensity for damage. Everything from muscle atrophy as we grow older to dementia in the elderly is at least partially a result of damage by free radicals. This same process very likely contributes to hormonal decline as we age. Damage to our DNA from continual exposure to free radicals almost certainly plays a role in the development of cancer. **Estimates suggest that the DNA within each cell in the body receives an average of 100 "hits" from free radicals each day.**

The good news is that our cells have very effective, innate repair mechanisms that have evolved over time. Enzymatic processes are constantly repairing breaks in DNA, repairing damaged machinery and filling in defects in cell membranes. These are the most basic healing functions of the body. Healing processes can, however, become overwhelmed by free radical production. Cell survival is very dependent on a diverse group of substances known as *anti-oxidants.* These chemicals have the ability to neutralize free radicals before they have an opportunity to damage vital elements of the cell. Cells have the ability to generate anti-oxidants, but dietary sources of anti-oxidants are also vitally important.

Free radical production is not limited to the inside of cells. Other types of free radicals can be found within the body. Free radicals are actually generated by cells of the immune system to do away with offending substances and invaders. This process occurs in the bloodstream and spaces between cells. It is a vital part of the healing systems of the body. A certain amount of this "inflammatory process" is in our best interest, but an exaggerated inflammatory response is a root cause of many diseases, from arthritis to atherosclerosis.

Free radicals can come directly from dietary sources. The most notorious of the dietary offenders, oxidized fat, is commonly found in processed food products of all types, processed meats, and food products that have become spoiled. Oxidized fats are especially concerning because they have the propensity to set off chain reactions in other fats, from cholesterol-containing lipoproteins in the bloodstream to cell membranes of all the cells in the body.

In the constant tug-of-war between these opposing forces, damage from free radicals always holds a little bit of an upper hand. This net balance in favor of free radical damage is termed *oxidative stress.* Oxidative stress is a potent force of disease. Minimizing oxidative stress is the key to slowing the process of aging. Fortunately for us, there are lots of different types of anti-oxidants, both naturally occurring inside the body and available from dietary sources.

Turning back our biological clock is impossible and oxidative stress is as much a part of life as breathing oxygen itself, but the burden of oxidative stress can be influenced by choice of diet and how we live our lives. Fresh vegetables and fruit are loaded with anti-oxidants and can definitely shift the balance in our favor. Unfortunately, only a minority of Americans take advantage of this simple opportunity to protect themselves from this significant factor in aging and disease. Even worse, the average American diet actually contributes to oxidative stress. Fats and oils used in processed foods, refined using high heat and chemicals, can become potent free radicals. That hotdog may taste good, but the contents are potentially deadly.

◊*Blood tests are now available to check your "anti-oxidant potential," but testing is rarely necessary for individuals following a healthy diet. An enormous variety of different anti-oxidants can be obtained from natural food sources. Testing for excessive inflammation in the bloodstream may, however, be worthwhile as it is a root cause of atherosclerosis. Ask your healthcare provider about having blood testing for "C-reactive protein."*

2 | TOXINS AND ALLERGENS

Well off the coast of Nova Scotia lies Sable Island, an isolated sand spit created by eddies between the Labrador Current and the Gulf Stream. At this remote outpost, a weather station monitors climatic changes and airborne toxins. Recently, <u>Cruising World</u> magazine featured a sailing trip to Sable Island. These quotes from the article poignantly illustrate the degree of concern we face as a culture:

> *"...on an island that seems so remote and pristine were instruments measuring ever-increasing levels of industrial aerosols, chemical insecticides and herbicides, methane, carbon dioxide, and other human-generated carcinogens, pollutants, and greenhouse gases."*

> *"Because of its location at the edge of the continent, Sable is in a unique location for making such measurements," stated the keeper of the station. "When the winds are easterly, we measure only traces of these substances. But when they blow from the west, well, then many of the measurements go off the scale, and Sable might as well be at the end of a huge, continental sewer pipe."*

Though some substances considered toxic to humans occur in nature, our world is gradually becoming saturated by toxic substances created by man. The conveniences of modern life have come with a price. The evolution of an industrial society has brought with it the introduction of an unprecedented amount of man-made chemicals into the environment, all having at least some potential for toxicity. Most sources suggest the list of man-made chemicals now tops 200,000, the majority of which were non-existent one hundred years ago. Initially, as man-made chemicals made their way into the air, the water, and across the surface of the land, it seemed the environment was like a huge sponge that could absorb it all, but eventually the level of toxins started to add up. We see it with fish kills along the coast, along with declining bird and amphibian populations worldwide, but there is little doubt that toxins in the environment also contribute to human disease.

In some respects we have become more "toxin aware" over the past fifty years, as open industrial waste-sites are less prevalent and many cities are making vigorous efforts to clean up their act, yet environmental toxins have become more pervasive than ever before. Our thirst for energy is high, and present regulations are not sufficient to protect the environment from pollutants released when millions of tons of coal are burned each year to produce electricity. Automobiles are designed to pollute less, but more people own cars and commute long distances. Chemical use in agriculture is still quite prevalent. *Everything* is made of plastic. Not only is the manufacture of plastics toxic, but plastics also leach toxins into the environment continually for a lifetime. Toxins of many varieties can be found in our food, in the water we drink and in the air we breathe...where we work, where we play, and in our homes.

Toxins have made their way into our environment insidiously. Rarely are concentrations of specific toxins high enough to be implicated in a specific disease process, yet common sense and a steadily rising cancer rate would suggest a cause for concern. We have come to accept toxins as being part of our everyday world, but our complacency means that the ever-increasing concentration of toxins in the environment is a real contributor to disease and adds up in ways that you would not expect.

When humans living in industrial areas of the world are randomly tested for toxins, the findings are alarming. A stew of chemicals including styrene (found in Styrofoam, plastic containers and computers), trichloroethylene (dry cleaning), dioxins (bleaching agents), PFC's (nonstick cookware), phthalates (plastic, vinyl, nail polish), PCB's, pesticides, xylene (plastics) and many others are routinely discovered. When laboratory animals are subjected to these chemicals individually, cancers and terrible diseases result—imagine the effect if they are all mixed together. (www.pollutioninpeople.org).

It is now common knowledge that larger fish such as swordfish are contaminated with mercury, but have you ever considered why? Certainly the ocean is not saturated with mercury, but it has to come from somewhere. Surprisingly, for fish in the Atlantic Ocean, the source is coal-fired power plants on the North American continent.

Coal is high in mercury. Mercury and many other pollutants carried in the smoke precipitate onto the land and are washed into estuaries by rain or precipitate directly onto the surface of the ocean. Micro-organisms take up the pollutants, and in turn, are eaten by larger animals. With each step up the food chain mercury is further concentrated in the animal's tissues. The cycle continues until the highest concentrations are found in the largest animals in the ocean. This food chain phenomenon is not limited to fish. Many airborne pollutants end up in our water and food supply via this mechanism. Toxins accumulate in fatty tissues of *all* animals, including and especially humans.

Toxic heavy metals including aluminum, antimony, beryllium, bismuth, cadmium, lead, mercury, thallium, uranium are much more prevalent in the environment today than ever before. Mining brings these elements to the surface from deep in the earth. Living organisms, having never been exposed to these elements to any significant degree, are at significant risk. Illnesses in children associated with exposure to lead and birth defects in newborns associated high levels of mercury in humans are cause for grave concern. Warning about consumption of certain fish is now a standard part of pre-conceptual counseling.

We deal with a similar phenomenon in agriculture. Chemicals used in agriculture are certainly toxic to pests and their use in production of grains, vegetables, and fruit should be of concern, but because concentrations of pesticide residue are not high, regulatory agencies such as the FDA suggest that traces of man-made chemicals found in our produce are not enough to worry about....but *should* we worry?

Most of the chemicals used in agriculture are fat soluble, and plants generally have very little fat. It is true that toxic chemicals mostly end up as a residue on the surface of the vegetable or present in small amounts within the oil-containing germ of grains. The actual measurable concentration of chemicals is low. Even so, environmental toxins found in our food are very real contributors to disease. The key to the concern lies in the fact that most toxic chemicals are fat soluble, and, even when consumed in minute amounts, these substances accumulate and concentrate within the fatty tissues of any living organism that consumes them. **The more fatty tissue, the higher the level of concern!**

Livestock and poultry fed a continuous diet of toxin-tainted grain, concentrate these subtle amounts of chemicals into their fatty tissues. Mostly confined to tight quarters with little ability to move around, these animals have a higher tendency to retain toxins. Hormones, which are also fat soluble, are widely used in this industry. The result is meat that is excessively fatty and may contain concerning levels of toxic chemicals. Often these chemicals are hormonally active. Humans, being right up there at the top of the food chain, in essence get a double dose of toxins when they consume meat from animals raised in this fashion.

Ever wonder about the association between breast cancer and consumption of red meat? Think about it: any toxins or hormonally active substances found in the fat of that nice juicy hamburger or steak are further concentrated in the fatty tissues of the individual consuming it. Hormonally sensitive breast tissue is predominantly fat and that's where toxins may end up.

Most of the time the role toxins play in chronic disease is only a piece of the puzzle, but occasionally it can be a major factor. Not infrequently, I have been able to provide direction and hope to individuals with chronic disease just by asking questions that others had not asked. I can remember one patient who owned a cleaning business and was exposed to potent chlorinated chemicals on a daily basis. Chronic fatigue and chronic sinus infections had developed insidiously over several years. She had been through the gamut of antibiotics, anti-inflammatory medications, and antihistamines with a progressively worsening condition. While seeing her for a routine exam, I suggested that avoiding chemical exposure was the only way she would ever get well. A complete lifestyle change is a tough recommendation, but after several years of no improvement, she finally sold the business. Once free of the toxins, her symptoms gradually resolved completely.

There have been numerous patients since then: the farmer with chronic sinus abscesses who was regularly exposed to chemical pesticides; a manicurist who spent her days inhaling nail polish and could not get rid of vaginal yeast infections; and numerous patients with headaches and other odd complaints who work in retail businesses where the air is always saturated with the smell of plastic. None of them had had improvement with conventional medical therapy. Resolution of these problems could only be expected with removal of the inciting factors. We would all do well to be more "toxin aware," as sometimes even the most blatant sources of toxins do not seem so obvious.

Exposure to toxins is sometimes self-inflicted. Smoking cigarettes and chewing tobacco are at top on the list. Alcohol is definitely a toxin (admittedly, in moderate amounts this toxic effect seems to be balanced by other, beneficial ingredients in wine and beer.) It goes without saying that illicit street drugs are harmful. Though pharmaceuticals are delivered in non-toxic and often beneficial doses, most have the potential for toxicity. Many, if not most drugs poison enzymes in the body to achieve a desired result. *All* drugs have the potential for side effects. Many drugs have the potential for tolerance, dependence, and withdrawal syndromes. Ironically, many drugs used therapeutically for treatment of chronic disease are known to suppress the immune system, certainly not in keeping with an intended goal of therapy meant to improve health.

Often the only difference between a beneficial drug and a toxin is the dose. Therapeutic medications have great value, but their potential for toxicity must be respected.

Because toxins come from so many diverse sources, they exert their negative effects in different ways. All biochemical reactions within the body can be, in effect, "poisoned" by different toxins. Toxins can directly damage DNA. Some toxins generate free radicals or are free radicals themselves, increasing our burden of oxidative stress. This is a major factor in diseases such as atherosclerosis and arthritis. Many toxins derived from pesticides and plastics have the potential to mimic hormones in the human body, providing a direct link to hormonally active cancers such as breast, uterine and prostate.

It is estimated that at least half of man-made toxins have the ability to affect hormone systems in the human body in some way.

Occasionally, as in the case of therapeutic drugs, these effects are desirable, but most often they are unwanted or harmful. Toxins tax the healing systems of the body and cause damage to the immune system allowing increased susceptibility to disease. The effects are subtle, but cumulative over time; measuring the exact contribution toxins make to disease is virtually impossible.

Fortunately for us, the body does have the ability to eliminate toxins via a very sophisticated detoxification system. As we have come to know, most toxins are fat soluble. To be eliminated by the kidneys and intestinal tract they must be converted into water soluble substances. This process occurs almost exclusively in the liver. Eliminating toxins is dirty business. The detoxification process produces free radicals that over time cause damage to the cells of the liver. As we age, this affects not only our ability to remove toxins, but other functions of the liver as well.

Be kind to your liver. Become more "toxin aware" by minimizing everyday sources of toxins. Not smoking cigarettes and acquiring adequate protection from occupational exposure to toxins goes without saying. Regular consumption of antioxidants provided by a diet high in fresh vegetables and fruit helps protect liver function. Vegetables from the cruciferous family such as cabbage and broccoli are especially protective of liver function. Dietary fiber provided by vegetables, fruit and whole grains is essential for adequate toxin removal. Drinking plenty of water helps flush things through. Exercise facilitates removal of toxins via increased blood flow and sweat is a route of elimination for some toxins.

◊ *Testing for a number of different types of toxins via hair samples or blood tests is available and can be considered by individuals with chronic disease or who have higher than average exposure. Testing for heavy metals is also available, but the testing is more complex. Individuals retain toxins differently depending upon the person's genetics, liver function and amount of body fat.*

ALLERGENS

Allergens can be simply defined as substances that induce allergic reactions. Allergic reactions are hyper-reactive responses of the immune system, causing symptoms. People can have allergic reactions to many different substances. Substances defined as allergens are generally nontoxic to the majority of individuals, who lack sensitivity to that substance. In contrast, toxins are substances that cause harm to *all* living things, to one degree or another.

Types of allergies and the degree of reactions vary widely. The most common allergic reactions occur to airborne substances such as dust, mold, pollen, and animal dander. Allergic reactions of the skin can be manifested directly (as with poison ivy) or can be a reflection of an internal allergic response (as in the case of a drug reaction or a bee sting). Typical symptoms of allergic reactions include watery eyes, runny nose, sneezing, itching and swelling of the skin and mucous membranes. Severe reactions include difficulty breathing and shock. Onset of symptoms associated with an allergic reaction is immediate.

Allergic reactions to foods can be severe, but true food allergies are not actually all that common. True food allergies must be differentiated from food sensitivities, which are relatively common. Food sensitivities are generally associated with gastrointestinal dysfunction and immune hyper-stimulation. Typically, multiple foods are involved. Unlike symptoms of true allergy which are immediate, symptoms of food sensitivities are highly variable, nonspecific and generally delayed for hours or even days from the time the food is consumed.

Almost anything can cause an allergic reaction. Everyone has allergies to something. Mine is a most convenient allergy—contact of my skin with raw shrimp causes an immediate and intense allergic reaction with itching and swelling, but as long as someone else heads, peels, cleans, and cooks them for me, I can eat all I want. My son's allergy is even more convenient— his reaction to poison ivy is severe enough to get him out of most of the yard work.

In some rare individuals, allergies can be life-threatening. Even brief exposure can mean a trip to the hospital or death. For most individuals, however, allergies are a non-life-threatening irritation. In average people, allergies become a significant problem only when the immune system becomes dysfunctional. Other factors of disease including poor diet, toxins, stress and microbes can contribute to immune dysfunction. Immune dysfunction contributes to other disease processes such as atherosclerosis and arthritis—everything is interrelated.

◊*The obvious way to avoid an allergic reaction is by avoiding the offending allergen, but when the immune system is in a hyper-reactive state, exposure to a single trigger can set off a cascade of reactions. Allergy testing can be beneficial for identifying specific allergens, but better health practices in general are beneficial for calming a hyper-stimulated immune system and reducing the intensity and frequency of allergic reactions.*

3 | POOR NUTRITION

You can tell a lot about a person's health just by examining what he or she eats. As much as the wrong foods can cause ill health, the right foods can be protective from damage resulting from other factors of disease. Ironically, here in one of the wealthiest countries on the planet, many (if not most) people are suffering from malnutrition. Not the protein-deficiency malnutrition found in the third world, but a form that is self-imposed. The prefix "mal" literally translates to mean "bad" and the types of "bad" nutrition that we suffer from result mainly from excesses rather than deficiencies. The average American diet contains gross excesses of starch, sugar and abnormal fat. This shift in balance caused by industrial-scale processing of food occurs at the expense of fiber and nutrients found in natural foods that are so vital for good health.

When it comes to food, you can almost think of it as being living or dead. Living food, as you would expect, appears in its original form—a stick of broccoli, a carrot or fresh shrimp. Living food provides for much more than a source of energy. Minerals, fiber, healthy fats, natural enzymes and all of the nutrients essential for good health can be found in forms that are easily and naturally assimilated by the body. These vital nutrients are hard to duplicate.

A tasteless, hard pear, if left in the windowsill long enough, will ripen into a soft, sweet delicacy. During ripening, the deeper flesh is protected from oxidation by the tough outer skin. Ripening occurs as enzymes present in the fruit break down the hard tissue into sugar. When we consume the pear, natural enzymes aid digestion.

There are many types of enzymes present in different types of living food. Beyond digestion, the body has the ability to absorb certain enzymes for use in other ways. Enzymes that break down proteins, called proteases, have anti-inflammatory properties and may protect against atherosclerosis. Processed food is totally devoid of natural enzymes.

All the qualities that make living food desirable (highly absorbable nutrients, just the right balance of sugars and favorable fats, antioxidants and digestive enzymes) also make living food highly susceptible to spoilage. Food preservation, especially when it includes chemical preservatives, decreases the nutritional value of food. Living food is best when consumed at the peak of freshness. Fortunately, we live in a time when fresh food is more available than ever before.

The average American diet contains little food that resembles its natural origins. Food that has been pounded, pulverized, over-cooked and over-processed could certainly be classified as dead. Dead food has no resemblance to the original food source and almost exclusively comes in a synthetically derived form—always with an over-abundance of starch, sugar and fat, designed only to appeal to our senses of smell and taste. If there are any significant nutrients present, they are usually synthetically derived additives that never match the nutrient potential of real food. Most often this type of food comes in a package or a box that is also designed to appeal to our senses.

"Factory farms" and industrial food production could easily be targeted as the source of our dietary woes, but we can only blame ourselves. The commercial food industry only gives us what we want. We have a natural craving for foods that are high in sugar and fat because the immediate need for energy is preferential over other nutritional requirements. This is quite a change from how it has been for most of human history. For many thousands of years humans were relegated to a very high fiber, high nutrient, low energy diet—not by choice, but by availability. With the advent of choice, our natural cravings pushed us to consume a diet very in high energy, but otherwise deficient in vital nutrients and fiber.

Reliance on high-energy, processed foods is the root cause of the American epidemic of obesity that has evolved over the past fifty years. Excessive body fat is associated with increased risk of heart disease, increased wear and tear on joints and ligaments, increased risk of certain types of cancer and increased risk of chronic disease in general. Often "central" obesity is accompanied by an alarming collection of signs and symptoms including *elevated fasting blood glucose, hypertension, decreased HDL cholesterol and increased blood triglycerides.* This condition, referred to as *insulin resistance syndrome, metabolic syndrome* or *syndrome X,* now affects somewhere between 25% and 50% of the population.

Obesity, once established, is not an easy problem to overcome. The first and most important goal in any successful weight-loss strategy is regaining lost health. The advice and guidelines in this book are designed to address this primary goal. Actual weight loss will occur gradually over time just by staying with good health practices. The weight loss process can be augmented with therapy designed to rectify hormonal imbalances and increase metabolism. For optimal results, therapy should be directed by a qualified healthcare provider. In cases of extreme obesity surgical procedures may be indicated and can be life-enhancing.

The shift in our food supply has occurred within a period of only a hundred years—almost overnight in relative terms, and certainly not enough time for the human body to adapt to such a drastic change. Though it is more convenient for a busy American lifestyle, the overall costs in terms of human health are enormous. Our total healthcare expenditure would be dramatically reduced if the American populace simply started making better food choices.

An ideal diet should consist predominantly of whole vegetables and rounded out with a variety of whole seeds (grains, nuts, and beans), whole fruits, free-range meats, seafood, and carefully chosen oils. Better choices in food slow the absorption of glucose, strengthen cell membranes, decrease inflammation, provide fiber for optimal digestion and toxin removal, and provide for optimal nutrients and minerals. Though most Americans are regularly making poor food choices, good food choices are more available than ever before. We are truly living in the "Golden age of food"—if you take the time to look for it.

4 | EMOTIONAL STRESS

It was the first day of summer when Mary returned with a chronic cough. She had been battling respiratory infections through the winter and spring, receiving numerous courses of antibiotics. With each course of antibiotics she would come down with a vaginal yeast infection and come to see me. "Why do I keep getting this stuff?" she complained. Her evaluation had so far had included a normal chest X-ray and a negative tuberculosis test. Allergies did not seem to be a factor and I could not ascertain that she had been exposed an unusual burden of toxins. Something was, however, having an adverse effect on her immune system and my next question brought out the reason. When asked how much she was sleeping, she answered, "about five hours on a good night." Emotionally it had been a terrible year for her and she rated her stress level as being extremely high. When these issues were addressed her condition gradually began to improve.

Day-to-day living causes a certain amount of emotional stress that is not detrimental from a health point of view. Stress can be a motivational factor that gets us going on to the next thing in life. Emotional stress only becomes a problem when it begins to rob the healing potential of the body. For many individuals this is every day. Well recognized as the root of anxiety and depression, emotional stress can aggravate virtually all disease processes. When patients ask if emotional stress could be playing a role in their particular problem, my answer is always a definitive "yes." Understanding and managing stress is an important adjunct in the treatment of *all* diseases.

For simplification, we can think of the body as having an "alert mode" and a "healing mode." Classically, the "alert mode" would be induced by a confrontation or threat such as having a dog run out in front of your car. With a surge of adrenaline, pulse quickens, eyes become wide, breathing rate increases, and muscles tense. All resources of the body are directed toward dealing with that threat. Other general maintenance functions, such as digesting food, normal immune functions, and daily maintenance and repair are placed on hold. Assuming the brakes work and the dog is fast, the threat passes, the mind relaxes, and the body goes back to normal affairs.

In an average American life, however, confrontations of some sort are seemingly a minute-by-minute affair. We never get a break. Excessive daily stress constantly places us in alert mode and prevents day-to-day repair and maintenance from occurring. The link between stress and diseases such as hypertension, autoimmune diseases, atherosclerosis and even cancer should be obvious. With a stressful lifestyle, we unknowingly place normal gastrointestinal function at a level of low priority while at the same time bolting down unhealthy food on the run. Is it any wonder that drugs for gastro-intestinal maladies are some of the best-sellers on pharmacy shelves?

The body is continually in the process of damage control and general maintenance, but it needs resources to do so. The energy and resources of the body are most devoted toward healing when they are not taxed in other ways. This "healing mode," as I like to refer to it, occurs when the body and mind are completely relaxed. Healing occurs most intensely during deeper stages of sleep. As we age, chronic disruptions in hormonal systems prevent the body from relaxing properly and sleep becomes less efficient.

Ironically, at a time in life when we would seem to need sleep the most, restful sleep is hard to gain. Learning tools to encourage spontaneous relaxation of the body and the mind become immensely important as we age.

5 | PHYSICAL STRESS

Another type of stress that is part of day-to-day life is basic *wear and tear.* The daily grinding down of bones, joints, and teeth is to a certain extent unavoidable, but here again, there are ways to lessen some of the impact. First and foremost, staying at a healthy weight prevents undue stress on joints and ligaments. A healthy diet certainly contributes to maintaining healthy joints, ligaments, and bones. The right combination of dietary fats can actually decrease the inflammation of joints associated with arthritis. Exercise done appropriately with proper stretching ahead of time and practicing disciplines such as yoga lessen the effects of wear and tear on the body.

Physical stress can tax the healing systems of the body as much as any other stress. Extremes in temperature can be quite debilitating. Excessive cold is something that few of us are threatened with today, but cold temperatures have been an ever present concern to those who have ventured toward the most northern and southern regions of the globe.

I have always been fascinated with the story of Ernest Shackleton, who, in 1914, set out with a crew of 28 men on an attempt to cross the Antarctic continent by dogsled. Early on, their ship was trapped in an ice flow and crushed. The band of intrepid adventurers spent nine months moving with the ice flow until they escaped to desolate Elephant Island via three remaining lifeboats. Shackleton, with a crew of five men, sailed one of the lifeboats across 800 miles of inhospitable southern ocean to seek rescue. He survived the harrowing journey and returned months later to find all crew members alive.

Shackleton's adventure was one of a number of expeditions to the northern and southern poles that occurred during that time in history. What sets his experience apart was that the crew survived horrendous conditions for an astoundingly long period of time with no loss of life and minimal loss of limb. Different from other expeditions, they decided early on to supplement their food supply with seal blubber. Toward the end, this made up a large portion of their diet. Seal blubber contains very high amounts of omega-3 fatty acids, and I, for one, believe that diet was a key factor in their survival. Their blood was like antifreeze! Today the harvest of seals is appropriately banned and seal blubber probably contains much higher levels of toxins than it did in 1914, but regularly consuming other sources of omega 3 fatty acids certainly makes sense for many health reasons.

Most of us would rather be hot than cold, but extreme heat, especially dry heat can be quite threatening. Excessive heat and dehydration are becoming more of a concern as the world heats up. In 2003 Europe experienced the hottest summer on record. The loss of 35,000 lives could be attributed to either the heat itself or crop shortfalls associated with the drought. As the population of the world continues to expand and the atmosphere becomes hotter, severe heat waves and shortages of food production across the globe are something with which we will all have to contend.

Trauma, another physical stress, affects all of us during our lifetimes to one degree or another, but is less of a threat than in days gone by. Before about 1920, trauma was a major contributor to decreased life expectancy. Today, trauma and accidents are minor factors. As much as I would like to attribute this shift to people having better sense, we owe it all to "big brother." Rules, regulations, and government bureaucracies make us wear our seat belts, force manufacturers of automobiles and machines to make safer products, and in general, make our world a safer place. Even so, being ever careful and ever vigilant is a wise practice.

6 | MICROBES

Microbes rule the world. They always have and they always will. Historically, infectious diseases have caused more death and devastation over the years than war and all of the other causes of disease combined. Even today, infectious diseases are the leading cause of death worldwide. Modern antibiotics and vaccines have made inroads into cutting the loss of life, but this is chiefly in developed countries. The plague and the pox have given way to AIDS and influenza as causes of worldwide devastation. Gonorrhea, syphilis, and the common cold have never left us. Lyme disease is now widespread across North America and Europe.

Interestingly, the most successful microbes are not the most lethal. Success in the microbe world is defined by the ability to propagate and flourish. Killing or severely disabling the host can be counterproductive. Take your average common cold virus. The virus infects, propagates rapidly, and quickly spreads to another host before the initial host's immune system catches up with it. The minimally disabled host organism actively participates in viral spread. Cold viruses may be the most successful microbes on earth.

Though the production of vaccines in the late nineteenth century and effective antibiotics in the mid-twentieth century can be recognized as major contributors to increased life expectancy, we can mainly thank government bureaucracies and social services for the improved health we enjoy today. Improved sanitation and health standards have done more to protect us from infectious disease than anything else has. As much as I hate to sign over a portion of my paycheck every month to Uncle Sam, the cost of this part of our "social good" is worth paying.

A visit to a third world country is a real eye-opener. Well beyond the lack of funds to buy antibiotics and vaccines, the lack of sanitation and public health in third world countries translates into poor health for most of the population. Standards that we take for granted such as indoor plumbing, public restrooms, restaurant grading, and garbage collection are often rare. Health standards, in the way that we know them, do not exist. As a result, diseases such as cholera are still common. Tuberculosis and malaria are present now as much as ever before.

In developed countries, microbes have seemingly taken a back seat to other causes of disease, but be assured, they are still there—seen and unseen. Microbes contribute to disease in ways that you would not expect. There is strong evidence that diseases like juvenile-onset diabetes, multiple sclerosis, and cervical cancer are initiated by microbial infections compounded by malfunctions in the immune system. Many cases of chronic fatigue syndrome have been found to have an association with a history of Lyme disease and other microbial illnesses. Some speculate that all autoimmune diseases may have microbial origins.

Some of the most successful microbes are those that go unnoticed, and these "hidden microbes" are major contributors to disease. Again, the goal of a successful microbe is not to kill or even severely disable the host. They propagate and flourish in the background, producing chemical substances that inhibit or control the immune system and neurological system, all the while remaining completely concealed. To us, these chemical substances are toxins and though they make us feel miserable, they may not significantly shorten our lifespan. At some point we may find that many diseases have roots to microbes that are presently concealed from our detection.

As much as microbes can be the enemy, certain microbes are our allies in many ways. Favorable bacteria inhabiting our skin and internal passageways prevent infections from pathogenic microbes. We actually could not survive without the help of the normal flora of bacteria within our gastrointestinal tract. These bacteria aid in digestion, convert vitamins into active forms, and help us rid ourselves of toxins.

Poor dietary habits and overuse of antibiotics can contribute to overgrowth of pathologic strains of bacteria in places where we depend on friendly bacteria. Toxins produced by abnormal bacteria not only cause problems in the gastrointestinal tract but also have effects that are far reaching. In understanding this connection, it is not surprising to find studies that link excessive antibiotic use to breast cancer. Even diseases such as depression and autism have links to bowel function altered by bacterial imbalances.

Excessive use of antibiotics worldwide is contributing to the formation of "super-bugs," microbes that are not only antibiotic resistant, but also produce deadly toxins. Though overuse of antibiotics in human populations is contributing to the problem, a primary source of concern is use of antibiotics in agriculture. About 70% of antibiotic use occurs in the livestock industry. Because livestock are overcrowded and fed unnatural foods to fatten them up, they are often sickly. The "super-bugs" being created are gradually spreading into the broader community.

There are two main strategies for preventing disease caused by microbial infections: avoiding exposure and maintaining a healthy immune system. Accumulated knowledge of how bacteria, viruses, fungi, and parasites function allows us a better chance to avoid crossing paths, but complete avoidance is, of course, impossible. Our best chance of staying healthy in a world dominated by microbes is to keep our defenses up. Free radicals, toxins, and excessive stress tax the immune system. Good nutrition, regular exercise, and stress reduction best support a healthy immune system.

7 | ENERGY

$E=mc^2$, the common equation that defines that all matter is made of energy. We are beings of energy—most specifically a type of energy called electromagnetic energy. Our energy fields can actually be sensed by certain gifted individuals and are the basis of several forms of traditional medicine. Acupuncture uses well-placed needles in the skin and tissues to affect these energy fields in a positive way to rid us of certain symptoms. Modern medicine studies our energy fields for diagnosis of certain problems. An EKG measures the dynamic energy fields produced by the heart to diagnose many types of cardiac malfunction. An EEG machine measures electrical waves produced by the brain. An instrument called an MRI measures the electromagnetic energy of tissues to produce a picture of our internal organs. This unique technology is able to do this without causing any known damage.

MRI does not cause internal damage because electromagnetic energy is "non-ionizing." In other words, radiation from electromagnetic sources does not have the ability to strike and damage the internal components of our cells. Even so, a very difficult question to answer is how much our own energy fields are affected by energy fields around us. Most of us now exist in an environment saturated with conflicting sources of electromagnetic energy such as computers, hair dryers, and other electrical devices. How many times have you felt "out of sorts" after sitting beside a computer all day? The magnitude of this problem is unknown and difficult to evaluate, but probably does play a role in disease.

Other, more concerning forms of energy include X-rays, gamma rays, and UV rays. These types of radiation definitely have the ability to do damage to our tissues. Referred to as "ionizing" radiation, they act very much like free radicals. They have the ability to pass through the body and "hit" microscopic structures, causing damage. They also have the ability to create free radicals. Some forms of ionizing radiation such as X-rays and gamma rays can pass completely through the body, whereas, others such as UV radiation only pass "skin deep." Exposure to some ionizing radiation is unavoidable. We are constantly exposed to "background" radiation from the depths of the universe and from the sun.

The ionizing rays of the sun penetrate the skin and strike other molecules, generating free radicals. Free radical damage to cells and structures within the skin is a direct link to wrinkling, aging of the skin, and skin cancer. Sunscreen may be the best protection, but, surprisingly, a diet rich in anti-oxidants may be almost as valuable. I once heard a story about a fellow who had a habit of consuming a large container of juiced carrots and vegetables every day. They say he had a strange orange glow about him, but he was able to cruise the entire Caribbean in a small sailboat without a drop of sunscreen.

Exposure to some background radiation will always be unavoidable, but I wonder about how much effect nuclear testing and the use of nuclear reactors around the world have added to our daily exposure. As individuals we have very little say in the matter, but common sense would suggest that living within the vicinity of a nuclear power plant or a nuclear testing site would not be a wise choice. Supporting politicians who oppose nuclear testing also makes sense.

Some ionizing radiation comes from the earth. Most of it fits into the category of background radiation, which we can do nothing about. One type that all homeowners should be aware of, however, is radon gas. This radioactive gas is emitted from the soil in some locations. The gas collects in basements and crawlspaces and can be a threat. Testing kits are commercially available and protecting yourself is a matter of installing a simple barrier. If you live in an area where radon gas is a problem, testing your home would be wise.

Concern over sun exposure is not enough to compel me to forgo a life outdoors. As with all things in life, there is a good and a bad side to sun exposure. Exposure to the rays of the sun means exposure to ionizing radiation, but sun exposure is necessary for vitamin D production and is well-recognized for its value in cultivating an increased sense of wellbeing. Vitamin D is not only important for strong bones, but is vital for many functions within the body, including a properly functioning immune system. Wintertime colds and flu may be as much related to decreased production of vitamin D from lack of exposure to sunshine as to indoor confinement with other people. As for me, I will drink my carrot juice, eat vegetables regularly, and have my days in the sun as often as I can get them.

◊*As we shun the sun and apply sunscreen liberally (sunscreen blocks as much as 95% of vitamin D production), many people may have insufficient levels of vitamin D. Many experts are recommending vitamin D levels at yearly physical exams, along with appropriate supplementation.*

GENETICS, THE DECIDING FACTOR
Anyone who has seen the size of an average medical textbook would be obligated to wonder how so many diseases could come from such a

short list of causes. The answer lies in our genes: Our individual genetic blueprints are so diversely different that an almost infinite number of diseases can come from a lifetime of exposure to a limited number of stress factors. This means that people vary in their susceptibility to different diseases. One person may consume flour and sugar for a lifetime and never develop diabetes, while another with the same diet will be destined to be on insulin by age fifty. Some people develop heart disease from smoking cigarettes and others will develop emphysema. Still, the list of causes is the same.

We each inherit a unique set of genes, different from any other set of genes that have ever existed (unless you are an identical twin, of course!). Our genes, however, are not perfect. They carry a mix of variations that have been passed down through the ages from all of our ancestors. Some of these "defects" may have actually been adaptations that worked very well for our ancient ancestors, but are of disadvantage in our modern world today. For example, individuals who rapidly absorb glucose and turn it into fat may have had ancestors who also had this trait and were, during lean times, resistant to starvation. **Good or bad, our genes are the cards we draw and how we play that hand is a matter of personal choice!**

Our genetic blueprint codes for all of the biochemical functions within the body. Because these functions are so remarkably complex, there is a significant amount of room for variability and error. Though we cannot change our genes, we can sometimes work around genetic defects.

We all have adaptations in our genes that affect our risk of disease, but good habits can often overcome "bad genes."

On a basic level, nutritional modifications can alleviate the risk of disease by addressing the biochemical restrictions introduced by these genes. For example, most Native Americans have innate intolerance to high glucose diets. For thousands of years their ancestors existed on food containing almost no sugar or grain; however, this population of people has very high rates of diabetes when exposed to the average diets of today. Respect for their genetic history would suggest that this population should always follow a very low-sugar diet similar to that of their ancestors.

Sometimes specific mutations occur in genes that affect the biochemistry of that individual. Some people are born with PKU disease, the inability to metabolize the amino acid phenylalanine. When exposed to dietary phenylalanine they develop neurological disturbances and epilepsy. Removal of dietary phenylalanine allows completely normal life. There are many other examples of similar types of genetic diseases that can be alleviated by understanding the genetic defect and others still that could be treated with nutritional changes if we better understood the underlying problem. Autism is a common affliction for which there is no known cure, but many patients respond positively to specific nutritional therapies.

The strategy of being able to turn on, turn off, or bypass completely certain genes through dietary changes, nutritional supplements or specifically designed drug therapy is very interesting science. This is the future of medicine. Newer and more targeted drugs that act at the level of the gene, as opposed to blocking biochemical reactions to impede symptoms, offer a whole new avenue in the treatment of disease.

In the future you may be able to walk into a clinic and have a blood test that defines your entire genetic profile; the risk for each disease laid out in black and white. Certainly knowing your personal risk of specific diseases would be beneficial, but if most diseases have the same origins, why wait until that information is available? No matter what our genetic background happens to be, the choices we make in life will determine how much we get out of life. We all have the choice of being healthy if we desire.

At this point you may be adding up a mental list of factors that may be contributing to your personal risk of chronic disease—if not, you should be. Everyone has a threshold for chronic disease, defined by exposure to the forces of disease and genetic makeup. Symptoms do not occur until that threshold is crossed. You may go for years without symptoms while cumulative damage is adding up, then, almost suddenly, symptoms occur—different symptoms, seemingly unrelated symptoms. You may find yourself searching for a diagnosis, but your ultimate health will depend on whether you search for causes.

CHOICES

In some ways illness can be thought of as a state of mind. We make choices that make us ill. We are driven to make these choices by learned behavior from observing those around us and by human nature itself. We must free ourselves from poor health choices and learn to make better choices. Only when we accept these choices as being a necessity of good health and better life can we experience all that life has to offer.

The forces of disease represent the obstacles that prevent us from having a full, happy, and disease free life. Freedom from these obstacles is achieved by making better choices.

What about Sarah, my patient with GI and other symptoms? As she began to change her thinking, her situation appeared in a different light. Sarah now felt reassured that she probably did not have some terrible illness and that she would be able to overcome her problem. With my encouragement, she decided to proceed with on-going evaluations with other physicians, just in case, but her approach was much calmer. Sarah was starting to see how important it was for her to start making her own choices. She understood that being well was simply a matter of choice. Now, with a motivated patient, I sent her out the door with more extensive information to read about the causes of disease and a lifestyle questionnaire to complete before her next visit.

VITAL PLAN

CHAPTER 4

Factors in Healing

A scan of Sarah's questionnaire quickly revealed the source of her original symptoms. Her diet mainly consisted of processed and packaged food eaten on the run, her general health habits were poor, and her stress management skills were terrible, even on good days. Problems with a difficult teenager, conflicts in her marriage, and coping with an unsatisfying job had left her in a state of constant anxiety.

Her stomach was the first to suffer. Perpetually being placed on standby by chronic stress, her GI tract was left in a state of dysfunction. Slow gastric emptying distended her stomach and allowed stomach acid to splash back up into the esophagus, causing constant burning in her throat. Compounding the problem, Sarah regularly ate foods that adversely affected the ability of her body to heal itself. The linings of the stomach and esophagus (called mucosa) began to break down, allowing the acid to do further damage. Ulceration was the result. Once ulcers are present, an infection commonly occurs with a bacterium called *H. pylori*. Many experts have concluded that stomach ulcers are caused by this bacterium, but we also know that many normal people carry these bacteria without having ulcers, suggesting that it is a secondary infection.

There seems to be a widely-held belief that stomach acid is the root of the problem and most conventional medical therapy is geared toward eliminating acid production completely. In the short term this strategy is effective. Healing of the mucosal lining occurs, but without addressing the original inciting factors, the medications have to be taken perpetually. Pharmaceutical companies are acutely aware of this fact, and competition for the newest and best acid-reducing medication is high.

Somewhere along the way, everyone seems to have neglected to remember that stomach acid has purpose. Without acid, proteins are not broken down properly and the initial stages of digestion are not activated. Foreign microbes pass through unharmed. Food stagnates along the tract and digestion becomes even more dysfunctional. Bacterial imbalances in the colon can occur, leaving the patient with symptoms of gaseous distention and constipation alternating with loose stools. The possibility that long term use of these medications may adversely affect bone density and risk of cardiovascular disease makes them even more concerning. Even though Sarah's reflux symptoms were kept in check, the longer she took this medication, the worse her other digestive symptoms became.

Sarah had noticed that after the colonoscopy her symptoms improved for several days. This was not a mere coincidence. Preparation for the procedure included two days of a liquid-only diet along with complete flushing of the gastrointestinal tract with laxatives. The flush expelled the buildup of toxin-producing bacteria in the colon. It took several days for overgrowths of abnormal bacteria to again occur. This is the same experience many people have after using "colon cleanse" products. These products do not remove toxins from the body as much as relieve bacterial overgrowth in the colon. Unless dietary habits are changed, the effects are usually transient. Overuse of laxative-containing products poses the risk of damage to the colon.

Sarah's treatment for anxiety was similarly shortsighted. The brain and nervous system include a delicate balance of inhibitory (calming) and stimulatory (exciting) chemical messengers called neurotransmitters. The high adrenaline associated with a stressful lifestyle, in a way, uses up the inhibitory neurotransmitters, leaving the nervous system in a state of perpetual excitation. The common name for this state of imbalance is anxiety.

Anxiety is often treated with a class of drugs called benzodiazepines. In this country, Xanax and Valium are the most commonly used brand names. These medications are extremely effective for treating anxiety, but only in the short term. They work by replacing the normal inhibitory neurotransmitters, thus setting the nervous system back in balance. Unfortunately, they also suppress synthesis of the natural calming chemicals of the nervous system. This results in the brain and nervous system becoming dependent on the drug to remain calm.

Compounding the problem is the fact that the body's normal response to a drug is to break it down. The liver recognizes any type of foreign chemical as being a toxin and produces enzymes to get rid of it. The longer a foreign chemical such as a drug is around, the more rapidly enzymes are made to eliminate it. As removal of the drug accelerates, the original symptoms being suppressed by the drug gradually return. This can occur with any type of medication, from anti-hypertensive medications to antihistamines. In the case of benzodiazepines, the brain and nervous system are left in a perpetually excited state. The situation often spins out of control and peculiar symptoms occur, such as the ones Sarah was experiencing.

When evaluating a patient like Sarah, I not only consider symptoms, but also routinely go down the list of stress factors that contribute to disease. Often specific modifications can be recommended that help the patient reduce offending stress factors and encourage healing. Sarah's situation appears less complex when broken down into categories of causes.

Emotional stress is the disease category that initiated her symptoms and catapulted her into her present condition. To achieve a full recovery, Sarah would have to expend a greater amount of effort learning better stress management skills. Stress combined with poor dietary and eating habits compromises gastric function and can lead to esophageal erosion. Stress may also cause acid production when food is not present in the stomach, resulting in mucosal damage to the stomach and esophagus.

Routinely eating processed food on the run added to her burden of oxidative stress and increased inflammation, adversely affecting immune system function and increasing her risk of all known diseases, including and especially cancer. As with many chronic conditions, poor diet is a major contributor to poor healing. Her eating habits did not necessarily create her problems, but compounded all of them.

In Sarah's case the drugs were actually causing most of her secondary symptoms. This is not uncommon. Side effects of medications often mimic symptoms of actual disease. Distinguishing between the two is sometimes challenging. In the case of benzodiazepines, stopping the medications suddenly causes worsening of the side effects, complicating the picture even further. All synthetic medications have the potential for side effects and many have the potential to suppress immune system function. While drug therapy is sometimes indicated and necessary, it usually represents a compromise in care. All synthetic drugs should be used judiciously.

I discussed other disease factors with Sarah. She had not been infected with any unusual microbe, it seemed, but toxins produced by bacterial imbalances within her gastrointestinal tract had certainly contributed to her symptoms. Regarding radiation, she would be classified as having only average exposure, but because of cell-phones, computers and the like, her exposure is higher than people living fifty years ago. As with all of us, her genes defined her susceptibility to disease. She appeared to be more sensitive than average to imbalances of her inhibitory neurotransmitters and she seemed to develop tolerance to medications very easily.

Once she understood what was going on, Sarah was very motivated to make changes in her life, but often change does not come easily. It would take over a year of hard work and effort for her to regain good health. The first step was placing her on a slow taper to discontinue the benzodiazepine medication. To counteract the negative effects of the medication and reduce her symptoms, she was started on several natural supplements that carried no risk of habituation. This helped her cope and facilitated coming off the medication.

When it came to a healthful diet, Sarah was starting at ground zero. For most individuals used to an average American diet consisting mainly of processed foods, healthy foods are downright unpalatable.

For Sarah, making changes to a better diet was a real challenge. Vegetables had never been much a part of her diet, and nothing tasted good unless it was sweet or coated in fat. In the beginning she had to force changes, but as her diet improved she realized that she felt better and, unexpectedly, the new foods actually began to taste "normal."

Along with better eating habits, Sarah was started on several supplements to protect the mucosal lining and encourage healing of her esophageal and stomach linings without disrupting the normal functions of the body. Nature often provides in ways that man cannot. Digestive enzymes were recommended to improve digestion of food. A probiotic supplement was initiated to reestablish the normal bacterial balance of the colon until yogurt and other fermented foods became dietary staples. With time, Sarah was able to taper and eventually stop the acid-reducing medication completely and her bowel function returned to normal.

An essential component of her recovery was learning better stress management skills. The anxiety she experienced every day was an impediment to getting off the benzodiazepine medication and a roadblock to better health in general. In our overmedicated, stressed-out world, this is a challenge for anyone. Regular exercise is a good place to start, as improved blood flow is good for everything, but Sarah would have to learn other skills that she could apply throughout the day. She took up yoga and worked one-on-one with an instructor who taught breathing and relaxation techniques. The relaxation training helped her learn to focus on the moment at hand and shield herself from the negativism of the world at large. All of these changes took time and she had to modify her schedule accordingly, but returning to her previous life was not an option.

As her health habits improved, so did her blood pressure. Most cases of what is commonly referred to as "essential" hypertension (implying that we do not know the causes) can be readily explained in simple terms. States of high adrenaline induced by chronic stress cause constriction of blood vessels and elevated heart rate. Poor diet usually plays a role, as insulin resistance contributes to derangements in adrenal hormone function (also being affected by stress) with the result of fluid imbalances and further constriction of blood vessels. Abnormal dietary fats contribute to inflammation in the bloodstream with consequential damage to blood vessel walls. Eventually, "hardening of the arteries" occurs and hypertension becomes irreversible. Fortunately, Sarah's condition had not progressed that far. In the end, she was able to stop the blood pressure medication and her blood glucose returned to normal.

After a year of concerted effort Sarah happily left the medications and all of her symptoms behind. Her energy level rebounded and she could get more done each day. Her life was far from being stress-free, but she could tolerate stress better with improved stress-management skills. She would never return to her old life. Interestingly, there were spin-offs that she did not expect. Her husband stopped smoking and improved his eating habits. Their relationship became more amiable and family relationships in general improved. Beyond achieving better health, *she restored joy in her life!*

Sarah was lucky. She regained her health before reaching the point of finding a diagnosis. Her situation was relatively simple and intervention came early. Others are not so lucky. Sometimes cumulative damage has progressed to the point of a well-defined disease process and conventional therapy in the form of pharmaceuticals or surgery is mandatory. Even so, the kinds of changes that Sarah was willing to pursue should be first-line therapy for any disease process.

The body has an amazing propensity to heal itself, if given the opportunity. Doctors do not heal. Drugs do not heal. Only the body can heal itself.

Sometimes doctors do have an opportunity to point the body in the right direction, *but true healing can only come from within.* The first responsibility of any healthcare provider is to help the patient create a healing environment by providing information and therapies that promote healing. A part of this process may include alleviating symptoms and correcting hormonal imbalances with conventional medicines and alternative therapies, but the urge to go for the "quick fix" should be resisted. Therapies should always be directed toward helping the patient actually heal.

As a surgeon, I am frequently humbled by the realization that my skills and training would be nothing without the profound healing potential of the human body. Almost as soon as an incision is made, healing begins. Bleeding dries up almost as quickly as it started. The immune system works overtime to eradicate any microbes that have inevitably slipped through the "sterile field." The liver immediately detoxifies any drugs used to induce anesthesia. Before the procedure is finished the body begins to adapt to whatever changes have been made. By the next day the incision has sealed over. By one or two weeks later the patient is well on the way to recovery. All of this is of course quite dependent on the ability of the body to heal itself. The success or failure of a surgery is generally much less dependent on the skills of the surgeon than on the overall state of the patient's healing systems.

THE HEALING SYSTEMS OF THE BODY, IN BRIEF

Healing begins at a microscopic level within each and every living cell. Repair mechanisms are constantly at work rectifying damage caused by free radicals and toxins to DNA and other functional parts of the cell. Most of the time, equilibrium is reached and the cell remains viable, but sometimes cumulative damage is overwhelming and the cell begins to function improperly. At this point the cell must "auto-destruct" before it begins the abnormal growth process that we know as cancer.

Our immune system is responsible for recognizing and obliterating these abnormal cells. Collectively, the immune system is the most elaborate part of our healing system. Not only is it responsible for scavenging potential cancer cells, but it also collects cells that are simply worn out and protects us from foreign invaders such as microbes or toxic substances. The immune system is composed of a complex network of cells and chemical messengers. It also includes the detoxification systems of the liver and the spleen. When everything is functioning properly, we go about our business in good health, totally unaware that our existence is being relentlessly threatened.

Much of disease occurs because the immune system is overwhelmed or has malfunctioned. Even though malfunctions in the immune system can occasionally be traced to specific genetic defects, most of the time the causes are environmental. All of the known factors of disease—nutritional deficiencies, excessive glucose and abnormal fats, oxidative stress, toxins, emotional and physical stress, microbes and radiation—play a role in adversely affecting immune function. **Though we cannot change our genes, we definitely have a say in controlling our exposure to these other primary factors.**

Dysfunction in the immune system can be manifested in several ways. Mobilization of the cells and chemicals of the immune system is part of the normal healing process. When this process is excessive and damaging, it is termed inflammation. *Chronic inflammation** is one of the main processes of disease. This exaggerated immune response is the basis of everything from arthritis to heart attacks and strokes. Chronic allergies also result from a hyperactive immune system. A malfunctioning immune system can turn on us and attack our own tissues in various ways resulting in a class of diseases referred to as the "autoimmune diseases"—but the most concerning malfunction of all is, of course, cancer.

I've heard it said that cancer is cause for concern and everything else is just an inconvenience. To some extent this statement is very accurate. Cancer is the diagnosis that nobody wants. Cancer is more threatening than any other disease process and despite all the money that has been poured into cancer research; we are still in the dark ages when it comes to treatment.

I wish I could tell you that adopting a better diet and a healthier lifestyle would alone cure cancer, but life is never quite so simple. These factors can certainly help prevent cancer, but cannot alone provide a cure once cancer is established. Two basic things have to happen for cancer to occur. First, cells in the body have to become mutated in such a way that they become abnormal and their growth becomes unrestricted. This actually happens all the time, but one of the primary jobs of the immune system is to recognize these cells as being abnormal and remove them. The real problem occurs when a flaw in the immune system continues to recognize these abnormal cells as normal or "self" and their growth continues uninhibited. Once established, this process is hard to reverse.

Once a cancer is established, improved health practices are not enough alone to cure the cancer, but they are essential for helping the body heal and also are important for helping the patient survive therapy. Presently, the

---

* I am sometimes asked why inflammation is not listed as a cause of disease. The answer is a simple matter of cause and effect. Inflammation occurs as a result of the factors of disease and is therefore a process or manifestation of disease and not a cause in itself.

only effective therapies for cancer are surgical excision, chemotherapy, and radiation—all therapies that are potentially toxic to normal tissues as well as to the cancer. Improved health habits and detoxification are as important for surviving the therapy as the cancer. Any strategy for overcoming cancer should include comprehensive health revitalization.

None of the modalities for treating cancer available today are ideal and hopefully the future will provide clues of how to repair the immune system malfunction itself. Until then, the best strategy for dealing with cancer is prevention. With the majority of our resources focused on early detection and finding "the" cure for cancer, a superb opportunity for prevention is being missed. **In my opinion, if we devoted a decent portion of cancer research funding toward educating the public about preventative measures, we could decrease the rate of cancer by 50% or more!**

THE COAGULATION SYSTEM

Closely tied to the immune system is the coagulation system, the healing mechanism responsible for tissue repair. When we are injured, an elaborate sequence of chemical messengers and chemical cascades is initiated to clot blood, prevent bleeding, and begin mending of tissues. An excessive or abnormal response from the coagulation system can lead to abnormal clotting. Excessive coagulation is a contributing factor to heart attacks and strokes and is a risk factor for the formation of blood clots in the lower extremities. Heredity does play a role, but is far from being the exclusive cause. **As the saying goes: genetics loads the gun, but choices in diet and lifestyle pull the trigger.** The end of the smoking gun, not infrequently, is a cigarette; but poor dietary habits are also central to the problem.

Stress contributes to atherosclerosis through effects on the coagulation system. Chronic emotional stress causes platelets, one of the main components of the coagulation system, to become extra "sticky." Increased platelet "clumping" accelerates plaque formation. Stress management and natural "blood thinners" such as omega 3 essential fatty acids and garlic are important therapeutic additions to counteract this effect.

◊*Some people are "hyper-coagulators" and are at risk of thrombotic events (blood clots). Screening labs for genetic susceptibility include Leiden factor V, homocysteine, protein C deficiency, protein S deficiency and antithrombin.*

These tests should be considered in anyone with a family history of thrombotic events, especially if estrogen products are being considered.

HORMONE AND MESSENGER SYSTEMS OF THE BODY

The immune system, and all functions within the human body for that matter, could not function properly if all the different types of cells were going about their business independently. Synchronization of function requires elaborate communication systems which include the nervous system and hormonal systems of the body, cumulatively referred to as the neuro-endocrine system. Communication among the different systems of the body is essential for normal function, as a whole, and for healing to take place. These communication systems are so complex that we still do not completely understand them. What we do understand, however, is how easily they can become imbalanced.

Patients frequently ask to have their hormone levels checked, being quite sure the symptoms they are having must be related to some hormone being "out of whack." Often they are right on track, but do not realize that there are literally thousands of different types of chemical messengers in the body, and they are all interrelated. Even measuring something as seemingly straightforward as a thyroid hormone level is fraught with different interpretations by various experts and labs. Second-guessing and micromanaging these imbalances is challenging for even the best specialists in the field.

Central to the neurological and hormonal systems of the body is the hypothalamic-pituitary-endocrine connection (often called the Hypothalamic-Pituitary-Adrenal axis, HPA axis). If you strip away the thinking portion of the brain and leave only the reactive portions of the brain, this is what you have left. With the autonomic (automatic) nervous system, brain stem and peripheral nervous system included, it would be the near equivalent of the entire functioning brain, nervous system, and hormonal systems of a lower vertebrate such as a turtle. With only a limited portion of the brain devoted to higher thinking, a turtle can only respond to stimuli in a defined and predictable fashion. This portion of the brain and neuro-endocrine system allows the body to maintain balance in the face of constant change.

The *hypothalamus*, an almond sized structure at the base of the brain, and the autonomic nervous system together control body temperature, thirst, hunger, weight, glucose and fat metabolism, physical manifestations of mood, sleep, fatigue, night and day rhythms, blood pressure, heart rate, and gastrointestinal function. The hypothalamus can be thought of as the central thermostat of the body that maintains balance in the face of constant change. This balance is referred to as *homeostasis*.

Though small in size, the hypothalamus is central to all parts of the brain. It receives feedback from all of systems of the body, input from the sensory organs, and input from the higher thinking brain. Everything we think and feel influences the hypothalamus, and in turn, the hypothalamus influences all functions in the body. The hypothalamus exerts its influence by way of the *pituitary gland*, a small gland that hangs down from a stalk just below the hypothalamus. The pituitary gland, in response to hormones secreted from the hypothalamus, secretes hormones that regulate the *thyroid gland*, the outer portion of the *adrenal glands* (located on top of the kidneys), and the *reproductive glands* (ovaries and testes). The pituitary gland also regulates the balance of fluids within the body, stimulates uterine contractions in labor, induces breast milk, and secretes growth hormone.

The *autonomic nervous system* includes the reflexive or automatic parts of the nervous system. Examples would include the regular beating of the heart or the processes of digestion, functions that are beyond voluntary control. It also has a direct connection to the middle part of the adrenal glands where *adrenaline* is secreted. Adrenaline is the chemical messenger that gets us going in response to acute stress. Increased adrenaline secretion causes increased heart and blood pressure, increased muscle contractions, and increased mental acuity associated with the classic "fight or flight" response.

Maintaining balance in the face of continual change is what health is all about. Any of the factors of disease (stress and negative thinking are very high on the list) has the ability to induce imbalances in the system, resulting in many symptoms of disease. As all parts of the system are intimately interlinked, isolating and treating dysfunction in only one part of the system is often not effectual. A thyroid disorder is rarely a thyroid disorder by itself. Menstrual irregularly is rarely a problem with the ovaries alone. Even the symptoms of menopause, associated with the cessation of estrogen production by the ovaries, are manifested through imbalances in the entire hypothalamic-pituitary-endocrine connection.

Hormonal dysfunction is not a *cause* of disease, but a *manifestation* of disease. Emotional stress, oxidative stress, excessive dietary glucose, abnormal fat, toxins, radiation and microbes are the primary causes of disease. When these forces are acting on the body as a whole, glandular function becomes compromised. When stress factors that cause disease are minimized, some rebound in glandular function can be expected. How much rebound occurs is highly dependent upon the gland. Possibly the most sensitive gland in the body is the thyroid gland. The thyroid gland, responsible for managing metabolism, can be affected by any chronic disease process—therefore, supporting thyroid function is important whenever thyroid function is abnormal, especially in the face of chronic disease.

◊*Traditionally, thyroid function has been evaluated indirectly by measuring thyroid stimulating hormone (TSH), produced by the pituitary gland to regulate thyroid function. A high TSH suggests inadequate thyroid function. Many practitioners also routinely measuring the active thyroid hormones, free T-4 and free T-3. Iodine, essential for normal thyroid function, is often deficient in average American diets and supplementation is sometimes important.*

The thyroid gland is very sensitive to the factors of disease. If you have been diagnosed with a thyroid disorder, or any other glandular dysfunction for that matter, hormonal replacement may be necessary, but reducing the factors that caused the problem in the first place is essential!

Adrenal function and the reproductive hormones can also be adversely affected by the forces that cause chronic disease. The adrenal gland can be thought of as "stress central," because the main hormones produced by the adrenal gland direct where resources of the body will be allocated during stress. During prolonged periods of excessive physical or emotional stress, adrenal function can become compromised and the whole body suffers. Rest from stress is the ultimate solution, but support of glandular function through supplementation is sometimes indicated. The fluctuating and rhythmic nature of these hormones, however, makes evaluation and supplementation very challenging.

Adrenal and reproductive hormones fluctuate throughout the day, and therefore are more difficult to assess than thyroid function. Blood samples only offer a "snapshot in time" and are only indicated in certain situations. Salivary hormone levels offer a more general assessment of function and can be used as a rough guide but are less accurate overall than blood levels. Salivary levels of cortisol, a primary adrenal hormone, are considered the most reliable of any salivary assessments and are typically measured four times within a 24-hour period. Salivary measurements of other adrenal and reproductive hormones are less reliable because blood hormone levels are much lower, but sometimes can be beneficial as an imprecise guide for therapy.

The exception to all rules is menopause. Menopause happens. Even with the best of health habits, menopause still happens. It is a natural process, but has the potential to adversely affect all of the hormonal systems of the body. The hormonal changes that occur at menopause with the normal and natural cessation of reproductive function often throw a monkey wrench into the body's entire hormonal balance. Menopause is especially devastating when it occurs abruptly with surgical removal of the ovaries. Though hot flashes, night sweats, mood changes, and insomnia are classic, almost any symptom that occurs at this point in a woman's life can be attributed to menopause. In almost all individuals these hormonal imbalances gradually equilibrate over time, but in very symptomatic individuals, nutritional and herbal therapies with properly dosed, bio-identical hormone therapy can be safe, effective, and sometimes almost lifesaving.

Many well-meaning healthcare providers have a tendency to micromanage illness. Treating only symptoms with specific targeted drug therapy is often ineffective and can actually be an impediment to healing. Correcting hormonal imbalances is important, but overzealous hormone supplementation can actually impede restoration of normal glandular function. The goal of therapy should be support of glandular function, not suppression by over-supplementation.

We know that certain hormones such as insulin and thyroid are essential for life and must be maintained at normal levels throughout life. Other hormones, including reproductive hormones, melatonin and growth hormone, gradually decline with age, even in healthy individuals. Certainly any hormone found to be below normal for age in a symptomatic individual should be considered for replacement therapy, but whether to adjust all hormones to the level of a youthful adult is a subject of great debate.

A complete understanding of the complexities of the healing systems of the body is not a necessity to maximize the body's healing potential. From the intricate mechanisms constantly repairing damage created by free radicals, background radiation and toxins at the cellular level all the way up to destruction of threatening microbes by the immune system, our healing systems are constantly on guard and at work. By taking steps to minimize the impact of the forces of disease while at the same time providing ideal working conditions and proper nutrients for all the healing systems of the body, we can create an environment of optimal healing.

ACHIEVING OPTIMAL WELLNESS AND LONGEVITY

The irreversible, cumulative damage that we call aging is an inevitable consequence of being alive, but we can slow down the process by adopting improved health habits. The rate at which aging occurs is partially dependent on an individual's genetic makeup, but in most cases is more dependent on the degree of exposure to the forces of disease, which are, of course, quite modifiable. Ideally I would say that the sooner you figure this out in life, the better, but these concepts are hard to get across to young people who are healthy. Most people do not start becoming concerned about their personal health until it starts to falter.

Most of us are not aware that cumulative damage is occurring until after age 40. After the age of 40, the guarantee of good health is less and less secure. It all adds up. Minor complaints such as tiredness, difficulty losing weight, or elevated blood pressure are just the early warning signs. Symptoms foretell that change is coming, whether you like it or not.

None of us really likes change, especially when it comes to our health, and so often we look for the easy way out. We would rather find a quick fix or "magic bullet" that makes everything just right again, without making very much personal effort. The quick fix may include a drug, a regimen of vitamins, an herbal remedy or tonic, something off the TV or internet or even a surgical procedure, but these efforts alone rarely bring true health, harmony, or happiness in life.

Like it or not, life is synonymous with change. Learning how to embrace change instead of resisting it is a key aspect of enjoying life. Cultivating an open mind and an open heart are the first steps. So often I see patients with changing or failing health for whom I know changes in diet and lifestyle are all that would be needed to completely rejuvenate their health, but resistance to lifestyle modifications remains a roadblock. They choose a quick fix for symptom relief as a first choice and never really get better.

Ironically, adapting to change and changing with change is the only way to slow down the inevitable and detrimental change that is associated with aging.

For anyone willing to make some compromises, there is hope! Much of the damage that has been accruing for years is reversible. Good health is available to anyone! The healing processes of the body are always there, just waiting to get back in the game.

Recognition is the first step in overcoming chronic disease. Once the factors that cause illness are defined, it becomes hard to ignore them. Even individuals who tend to resist change will find it hard to hold on to bad habits when these habits are recognized as an impediment to feeling well.

Our health and wellbeing are determined by the choices we make each day. The choices for creating an ideal healing environment are simple and straightforward, but not necessarily easy to master in the fast-paced world in which we live. Self-discipline and compromises are necessary. The degree of compromise will depend on the condition of the healing systems of the body. Individuals with established illness may have to be rigidly particular about their health practices for a while, but be reassured that no matter what the degree of compromise, the benefits of renewed health will allow you to live life to its fullest.

Changing to a healthier lifestyle should not be equated with misery. "Healthier" means changing to different habits, but the changes can be pleasant—it all depends on whether change is approached with a positive attitude. With a positive attitude, better dietary and lifestyle habits are immediately complemented by feeling better and enjoying life more.

Guidance from other knowledgeable individuals is encouraged for help and support along this pathway. *Any and all disease processes* can be positively affected by paying better attention to the choices we make!

COMPONENTS OF OPTIMAL HEALTH AND HEALING

The four primary components of health and healing include *proper nourishment, cleansing and protecting the body, achieving physical fitness*, and *synchronization of the body and mind*. A fifth component includes all aspects of modern healthcare. All of the categories are interrelated and dependent on each other. Attention to each is necessary to create an optimal environment for health and healing. At the heart of each category is the matter of personal choice. As we make better choices, we can expect to be not only healthier, but also more successful in life's endeavors and more satisfied with life in general.

NOURISH A healthy body cannot exist without proper nourishment. A diet high in fiber, nutrients, and minerals with just the right amount of sugar and the proper balance of fat is achieved by regularly consuming vegetables, whole seeds (grains, beans, and nuts), fruit, seafood, and meat raised in a healthy manner. There is little room in a healthy diet for commercially processed food.

PURIFY Good food only goes so far in protecting the body. Learning where toxins exist in the environment and limiting your exposure to them, adopting good personal hygiene habits for avoidance of microbial infections, and maintaining gastrointestinal health for internal cleansing are all part of an optimal health strategy.

ACTIVE Regular exercise is just one component of staying physically fit. Adopting an active lifestyle is an essential key to longevity.

CALM Regular practice of relaxation methods for stress reduction are an essential part of good health; when these forces are combined with exercises in brain synchrony, a powerful force of healing is created. Brain synchrony not only opens the door to wellness but is the key to happiness and harmony, in general.

ENHANCE The primary focus of healthcare should be complimentary and supportive. Medical, surgical and alternative therapies work best when directed toward reducing the pressures that cause disease and mending or compensating for cumulative damage. Treating symptoms is important, but should be a secondary and hopefully transient concern.

Cumulative damage to the body is inevitable and sooner or later we will all need extra help, in one form or another. Less invasive and micro-invasive surgery can not only be lifesaving, but also life rejuvenating. Well thought-out medical therapy using combinations of nutritional supplements and herbal therapies, combined with less toxic pharmaceutical therapy can support healing, improve longevity, and make life more pleasant in general. Alternative therapies such as acupuncture, massage therapy, yoga therapy, energy therapy, chiropractic care and others can promote healing and reduce the aches and pains that are part of being alive.

Conventional medicine tends to do a good job of taking care of the acutely ill, but does little to prevent chronic disease from occurring. Holistic providers and alternative healthcare providers do a better job of considering other factors of health, but still tend to retain control of the situation. To achieve optimal health and healing, you must take charge of your own well-being. No one is going to take as much interest in your health as you do. Even then, addressing only one pillar of health will not suffice. To achieve the balance of health that optimizes the healing potential of the body, all of the components must be addressed. Don't be caught in the "too little, too late" mode—start making changes now.

A PLAN FOR CHANGE

As you read the second half of this book, you will acquire the knowledge and skills necessary to cultivate a plan for change. In the next section, NOURISH, you will learn about all the reasons why you should change to a healthier diet and how eating better can be a life enhancing experience.

In our toxin-saturated world, becoming "toxin aware" is a good practice. The first chapter in PURIFY, offers practical advice for learning where hidden toxins exist and how to limit exposure. The second chapter discusses the elimination and detoxification processes and how these important facets of health can be optimized.

For many people, following a regular exercise routine and learning better stress management skills are significant hurdles to overcome. The last two main sections of the book, ACTIVE and CALM, are designed to help you incorporate these important aspects of health and healing into everyday life.

Be patient as you read—everything will come together. Lifestyle changes do not happen overnight. Willpower comes in spurts, as the never-ending rotation of diet and exercise fads attests. Try one thing for a while until it becomes routine and then shift to something else. It does take some work and effort, but new routines will become habits over time. Unlike fads, which fade with the night, good health habits will last you a lifetime. Even people who have a tendency to see change as daunting can usually overcome obstacles and achieve their full health potential if they try hard enough. Once change becomes the accepted norm, life is always better.

Though each section is addressed independently, they must come together in practice. The conclusion pulls all of the principles discussed in the four components into a workable strategy for getting the most out of health and life. Suggestions are also made for formulating a strategy to overcome any type of chronic disease, where the same principles apply but must be practiced much more stringently.

If you are reading this and have a chronic illness, I would strongly encourage pursuing a thorough evaluation with an experienced healthcare provider—sometimes identifying and treating specific problems can augment your recovery—but do not wait for a diagnosis before beginning therapy! Mastering the principles outlined in the next four sections is your best bet for actually overcoming chronic disease. Whether your goal is losing ten pounds or overcoming a major illness, following the advice in this book will improve your situation.

The material in this book is complemented by a website, www.vitalplan.com. The website is a resource for new information, guidelines for reaching optimal health and protocols for health restoration. Information contained in the book is the cornerstone of therapy to restore normal health. The website adds a dynamic component to information. All complement any evaluation and therapy offered by your healthcare provider. A guide to basic lab screening is included in the appendix of this book.

REFLECTIONS ON CHANGE

On a personal level, I have certainly had to come to grips with change and compromise as much as anybody else. Life is not easy and by nature comes with challenges, though sometimes the most difficult parts are the ones that make life most interesting. Without challenges, life would be boring. Making good choices and accepting change is the best way to deal with the challenges of life. For the most part, I have come to accept change and in many ways have come to actually enjoy change. Maybe this is what maturity is all about.

The compromises that have become necessary with age have become a part of who I am. Regaining lost health has sometimes required effort and determination, but retrospectively, even that was not so bad. Life is now more settled, and I am more centered in many ways. I expect there will be more challenges in the future, and I hope to accept them gracefully. Some years down the road a simple life with a light diet of rice and vegetables, low stress, regular exercise, and daily meditation may be something to look forward to.

As a physician, my approach to the practice of medicine and healing has also changed and matured. Teaching and motivating patients about how to change or improve their own health is much more satisfying to me than handing out prescriptions. I have hopes that conventional medicine will mature in a similar way, and I have faith that modern science will provide us with better therapies for many diseases, including cancer. I am optimistic that change is on the horizon...that pharmaceuticals will lean more toward optimizing the healing potential of the body, rather than just treating symptoms...that surgery will become more and more micro-invasive...that traditional will be used alongside conventional...and that legitimate alternative and natural therapies will become a part of mainstream healthcare.

The human body has an amazing potential for healing, if given the right opportunity. The pressures from the forces of disease are great. Release the pressures and the healing systems of the body will always respond.

Nourish

Nourishment is intimately tied to overall health. The first step in adopting a healthier lifestyle is adopting a healthier diet.

CHAPTER 5

Food…A Historical Perspective

One constant among all life forms is the need for nourishment. Nourishment, most commonly in the form we call food, includes not only fuel for energy, but also chemicals and minerals necessary for normal biochemical and physiologic functions of the body.

The first priority of survival for any living organism is obtaining adequate nourishment. Human history has been particularly influenced by this pursuit. Humans have been wandering around this planet for a surprisingly long period of time. Human habitation of the earth goes back much farther than written history. Fossil records and DNA analysis suggest that our species, *Homo sapiens*, has existed for at least 160,000 years. Appreciating how our distant ancient ancestors lived and what they ate to survive is essential for understanding the nature of many of the nutritional problems that we face today. Like it or not, we are all a function of how our species evolved.

Imagine the world about thirty thousand years ago. The North American continent would not yet have been populated, but some humans would have migrated out of Africa and into Europe and Asia. A typical pre-historic man probably looked like you or I except for being very short by our standards and much scruffier in appearance. Being human, he would not have had the prominent face and sloped brow of a Neanderthal, so commonly depicted as the average caveman. Very likely, his body was covered in scars, since life was hard for a prehistoric man. We would expect his skin to be dark in equatorial climates, but fitting him into any race category that we know today might be difficult.

The primary activity of humans of 30,000 years ago was collecting food. What a primitive man wanted from his food and what he actually got were two different things. Priorities of survival dictated the need for sources of energy to power the body and sources of protein to replace the daily turnover of amino acids. Primitive foods, however, were far from being high in energy. A prehistoric diet came packed with nutrients, minerals, and especially fiber but offered little in the way of sugars and fat; protein content was also minimal. Without these vital components of food, starvation was an ever-ominous threat. **The drive to acquire enough sugar, fat, and protein for survival was stronger than any other, even stronger than the drive for sex.**

If we wanted to duplicate a "primitive-man diet," it might go something like this: an enormous variety of edible vegetable matter, fruits, seeds, fungi and nuts would be available for consumption, but none of it would resemble any food that we are used to today. We would find most of the food to be bitter or tasteless, with almost no sugar or fat. Cultivation of grain would not come along for another 20,000 years. With the absence of refrigeration and food preservation as we know it today, a significant portion of the food would have been fermented or even spoiled. In fact, selective fermentation of food is an age-old method of preservation.

Nothing came in a package. Sauces, dressings, added sugar, or added fat, of course, did not exist. Dairy cows did not exist, and no one drank milk past early childhood. Oil for cooking and frying was unheard of. Wild honey might have been available as a natural sweetener—if one braved extracting it from the hive. Protein sources included an occasional bit of fish or a small mammal roasted on a spit, but this probably was not an everyday occurrence. The occasion of all the boys sitting around the campfire roasting rump of mastodon was probably quite rare; an event mostly practiced by our brutish cousins the Neanderthals. Bird eggs, in season, might have been on the menu.

All waking hours would be spent collecting enough food for basic survival. Exhaustion from the labor of it all would ensure a good night's sleep, night after night. In colder climates a primitive diet consisted mostly of animal sources, but in the warmer climates where most humans lived, vegetable matter was almost surely the most consistent food source.

Many plant substances are toxic and the fact that our primitive man knew which ones to pick was not by chance alone. Some knowledge was passed along from his parents and others in his group, but much of it was burned into his genes by thousands of years of natural selection. Plant substances that we consider food or use for medicinal purposes today are "familiar" and generally well accepted—in essence, humans have been practicing herbal medicine for all of history. In this light, it should not come as a surprise to find that overly processed foods are commonly associated with disease and that synthetic drugs are often associated with side effects.

You can tell a lot about what types of foods an animal should be eating by examining its teeth. A typical herbivore, such as a horse, will have a few teeth up front specially designed for pulling grass and leaves from plants, with the remaining teeth consisting of molars for grinding vegetable matter into a pulp. A dedicated carnivore, such as a wolf, will display predominantly teeth for cutting and shredding meat.

Humans are omnivores. Examination of an adult human mouth will demonstrate two sets of incisors and one set of canines, intended specifically for tearing meat. Two sets of premolars and three sets of molars (one set are wisdom teeth) are designed for chewing vegetable matter. If the ratio of the types of teeth are considered, a normal human diet should consist of about 2/3's vegetable matter and 1/3 meat.

Despite his instinctive knowledge of "safe" foods, our primitive man was primarily driven by the need for glucose and fat. If we brought a primitive man back today, he would immediately rush over to McDonalds like everybody else. There, as at most modern fast food restaurants and most groceries, he would find an abundance of the sugar and fat that were limited in his natural diet. The drive to consume these types of foods would be so strong that he would soon be overweight, lethargic, and in ill health like many people today. It would not be long before we would find him sitting in front of a television, wasting away the extra hours not needed for collecting food.

For the human body, glucose and fat are the primary fuels. Dietary proteins can also be used in a pinch, but are more readily suited for making up the structural components of the body than being used for producing energy. Of the three, glucose is the most important. Glucose, in the right amounts, is really good stuff. It provides instant energy. It burns cleanly with few by-products, making it the preferred fuel for the brain and muscles. **The fact that taste of sweet tickles our taste buds like nothing else is no coincidence!**

We like fat just about as much. The aroma of sizzling fat from a thick steak on the grill is hard to forsake. Fat, as an energy source, is not as versatile as glucose and does not burn quite as cleanly, but it provides all-important energy for low-end power and endurance. The muscles of the heart use predominantly free fats in the blood as fuel. The muscles of endurance athletes such as long distance runners will convert from burning predominantly glucose to burning predominantly fat fairly rapidly as exercise progresses. Fat is also necessary for producing heat and providing insulation in a colder climate. Our basic primitive man living in prehistoric Europe or North America would have needed good sources of fat for survival.

In our present time of overabundance, the simple fact that only a small amount of glucose and fat are necessary for survival creates a significant dietary conundrum. Maybe in another 50,000 years humans could evolve to live only off of high concentrations of sugar and fat alone, but that does not help us right now. Like it or not, we have a strong dependence on all the other stuff that came with our ancestral foods. Though they do not affect our taste buds in nearly the same way, dietary fiber, enzymes, proteins, vitamins, minerals, bacteria from fermented food, and the host of beneficial chemicals found in plants are just as vital for our survival and well-being as sugar and fat. **The human body cannot function normally without them.**

The fact that we tend to ignore all the dietary "extras" is not a simple oversight, but is a result of how food sources of the world changed over time. Eventually humans grew tired of roaming the planet looking for food and figured out how to cultivate grain. Grains had glucose, fat, protein, fiber, nutrients, and minerals all rolled into one food source. Grains could be stored for the winter and transported long distances. No more wandering. Food actually began to taste better as grains, vegetables and fruit were cultivated to have more sugar. No need for hunting, either: domesticated animals could be fed grain and kept in one location. Humans thrived. Civilizations sprang up. The world changed. History was written.

The cultivation of grain itself was not necessarily a bad thing, as whole grains are fairly well balanced with carbohydrate (including fiber), protein, a little bit of oil, and some vitamins and minerals. The problem came when entire cultures became dependent on a crop of grain as a primary food source. Inevitable blights, droughts, and insect infestations commonly caused mass starvation and disease, a threat still common in the world today.

In spite of these problems, the advantages of grain cultivation were too much to ignore, and grain gradually became the dominant food source of the world: wheat in Europe, rice in Asia, millet in Africa and, to a lesser extent, corn in the Americas were the predominant grains. Even though grain did provide higher concentrations of glucose than were found in primitive diets, over several thousand years, most cultures adapted to it. Interestingly, there have been pockets of cultures around the world that have existed without dependence on grain. Descendants from these groups of humans—namely Native Americans, peoples from many parts of Africa, and Aborigines in Australia—never acclimated to the higher levels of glucose found in a grain-based diet and consequently have high rates of diabetes when exposed to the typical processed-grain diets of today.

For several thousand years of recorded history the status of food changed very little, until about a hundred years ago with the onset of the processed food revolution. The catalyst that fueled this change was the discovery of the energy contained within petroleum. Shifting from plow and mule to tractors quickly altered the world's food production capacity. Suddenly food in the form of grain could be produced on a grand scale, the likes of which the world had never seen before. Petroleum also provided the means to transport large amounts of it to anywhere on the planet. North America became the bread basket of the world with production of staggering amounts of wheat and corn. The world changed again. Populations surged. Factories sprang up. The pace of life quickened, in America like nowhere else.

The pace of a new American lifestyle demanded food that was simple, easy to prepare, and cheap. Convenience became priority number one. The commercial food industry responded by lining the shelves and aisles of newly styled "supermarkets" with pre-processed and packaged foods. To improve efficiency and keep costs down, only a limited number of food sources were cultivated. Today, a surprisingly large proportion of our food comes predominantly from only two sources: wheat and corn. Industrial refinement and plant hybridization pushed efficiency in food production to the outer limits and at the same time catered to those all-important tastes for sweet and fat. The cost was nutrition, but no one seemed to notice because everything tasted good.

The food processing and packaging industry has been very skillful in presenting a seemingly wide variety of unique products all derived from a limited number of food sources. Expert marketing is the key. Often more care and concern are given to the outside packaging than the food inside. Products are designed to appeal to our senses, especially capitalizing on those preferential tastes for sweet and fat—**giving people what they want always sells better than giving them what they need.** Today, packaged food products are so prevalent that many Americans rarely eat anything that doesn't come from a box or a wrapper.

When it comes to processed food, no ingredients are more ubiquitous than the "threatening three:" *refined wheat flour, high fructose corn syrup,* and *partially hydrogenated oils*—all derived predominantly from wheat and corn sources. These same ingredients are found in most packaged food products found on grocery store shelves today and they dominate the fast food industry. We are eating the same stuff over and over again. A look at the ingredients label found on a typical packaged food product will typically reveal at least one of the "threatening three" as well as preservatives, flavorings, and possibly added vitamins or minerals, but not very much in the way of good nutrition.

To make matters even worse, the corn and wheat consumed today is not the same as the grains consumed by our ancestors.

Extensive hybridization, for the sole purpose of increased production yield, has dramatically altered the actual composition of the grains. Heavy on starch, these grains release glucose more rapidly, a major contributing factor to the present epidemic of obesity, insulin-resistance and diabetes.

The dramatic rise in diabetes and metabolic syndrome over the past one hundred years has closely paralleled the increased consumption of processed corn and wheat products worldwide.

At present, we have such an abundance of grain that we not only have enough to feed ourselves but we have plenty left over to feed animals. In fact, the *majority* of grain and soybean production in this country goes toward industrial-scale livestock production. Grain is the ingredient that makes meat so tantalizing to our taste buds. I can remember growing up when meat tenderizer and a sharp knife were essential parts of eating a steak. Today, a steak cuts like butter and melts in your mouth. That exquisite taste is the result of abundant saturated fat from a corn-fed (a.k.a. "grain-finished") animal which ate, in its last months, an unnatural diet. Beyond having an unhealthy amount of fat, toxins (from the corn) that become part of the fat constitute an even graver concern associated with commercially-produced meat. It provides much more taste appeal but may compromise your health.

Turning back the clock to a different time in food history would seem to be a wise choice, but going back to a purely "primitive" diet is not a necessary move for good health. I can remember as a Boy Scout being turned loose in the woods for "survival weekends" with only a knife and a canteen. After several days scavenging for the "bounty of nature," we were always ready for a trip to McDonald's. We quickly discovered that surviving on a primitive diet is a hard way to get by. When the average American diet of today is compared to the average human diet of 30,000 years ago, we find two opposite extremes. **What we really need is something in-between.**

While most people allow their food choices to be dominated by the commercial food industry, they neglect to observe that we are truly living in the golden age of food. Fresh, nutritious, whole foods are more available than ever before. In the middle of December, I have access to locally grown collards, broccoli, cabbage, and winter squash; I can also enjoy fresh blackberries and strawberries imported from more southern climates, oranges and grapefruits from Florida, and many other fresh foods from around the country and even around the world. Though I do subscribe to the practice of buying locally whenever possible, the privilege of being able to supplement local seasonal foods with those from other places would certainly suggest we are living in the middle of the "Garden of Eden."

Even as petroleum supplies begin to decline and the world changes again, we should be able to maintain our Garden of Eden indefinitely if we make intelligent choices. Foods that are being transported by truck and plane could be transported just as well by train for a fraction of the cost. Better methods of preservation, such as flash-freezing meats and seafood on site, will allow slower and more energy-wise methods of transport.

The advent of refrigeration and freezing has allowed the nutritional value of food to be retained longer without preservatives. We should not have to resort to traditional methods of meat preservation such as drying, salting or use of chemicals. Many people still have a taste for sausage, ham, and other preserved meats, but these foods are not healthy food choices and should be consumed sparingly, if at all.

Fresh foods are more available than ever before, but we can make wise and healthy choices even with preserved foods. A hundred years ago, canning fruits and vegetables was a necessary part of every summer and fall routine just to have enough food for the winter. Today, refrigeration and freezing have answered that concern, but canned foods do offer convenience and economy. Canning is practical and involves the lowest expenditure of energy. Food is least expensive at peak harvest and that low cost can be retained within a can. Though many foods lose nutritional value with canning, certain foods such as tomatoes, beans, certain fruits and fish do rather well in a can or a jar.

Cost containment can also be applied to most fruits by simply removing water. Because fruits are high in sugar, drying offers a satisfactory method of preservation. I, for one, enjoy dried blueberries, cranberries and cherries in my yogurt year-round, and my pasta primavera would not be the same without sun-dried tomatoes.

The difference between an unhealthy diet and a healthy diet is simply a matter of personal choice. Though evolution has left us with an insatiable appetite for sugar and fat coupled with a normal desire to consume significant quantities of food, it is possible not only to achieve but also to actually enjoy healthy dietary habits. Healthy food and, just as importantly, the knowledge to know what defines healthy food are more available than ever before.

The "golden age of food" is truly upon us. Why squander it by making poor food choices?

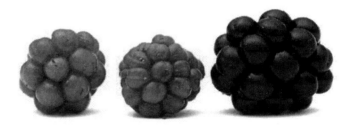

VITAL PLAN

CHAPTER 6

Food...A Scientific Perspective

The science behind food would have been of no interest to a primitive man. He did not take time to check labels for carbohydrate, fat and protein content; he simply ate anything that was edible, and as much of it as he could get. By necessity, he consumed a wide variety of foods, and his food came packed with vital nutrients, minerals and fiber. His greatest concern was obtaining enough glucose, fat and protein daily for basic survival. In the primitive world, acquiring energy from food trumped all other concerns.

If your diet consists of a wide variety of whole foods including vegetables, fruits, seeds, free-range meats, seafood, select dairy products and eggs, you may not be interested in the science behind your food, either, since your diet is contributing optimally to your health. On the other hand, if you were raised on a diet that included processed and packaged foods (as most of us born within the past seventy-five years have been), you may be interested to know how it has affected your health. Diseases such as diabetes, atherosclerosis and arthritis are directly related to diet and most specifically related to a processed-food diet.

CARBOHYDRATES

Carbohydrates include sugars and starches. Though there are many types of sugars in nature, the energy cycle common to plants and animals is built around the sugar glucose. This simple molecule makes life possible and while enough of it is essential, too much is a detriment to our health.

THE GLUCOSE PROBLEM

"Super-sized" American diets are super-saturated with glucose. The chief sources of excessive dietary glucose are starch and sugar found mostly in food products made from processed wheat and corn. From bread and bagels to donuts and pastries, processed wheat flour makes up a large portion of the food Americans consume on a daily basis—as for wheat, whole grain products are actually as bad as the white stuff. Modern wheat flour, white and whole grain alike, releases glucose faster than table sugar!

Starch, the main component of flour, is made of long chains of glucose linked together. By itself, starch is not very sweet; so many processed food products also contain some type of sweetener. Table sugar would do, but high fructose corn syrup is the sweetest of the sugars and is also the least expensive. The name is somewhat misleading, as it also contains a significant amount of glucose.

A simple concoction of flour, corn syrup, and fat tempts our taste buds like nothing else on earth—and with good reason! Of all the naturally occurring sugars in nature, glucose is preferred. Glucose is a very versatile fuel source. It burns cleanly with minimal free radical production and can be stored in the liver and muscles for immediate energy needs. Just as easily it can be converted into fat for long term energy storage needs. Glucose can also be utilized as a base for creating certain amino acids (the building blocks of proteins) and is an integral part of many of the components of a living cell.

Glucose is a metabolic "must-have," but something that you do not need very much of to be healthy. In fact, having more than necessary is actually very toxic.

The toxicity of glucose relates to its inherent tendency to stick to **proteins.** Like carbon deposits built up on the pistons and cylinders of your car's engine, glucose sticks to proteins and gums up the vital machinery of the human body. Performance is adversely affected. This cumulative phenomenon occurs in all of us and is a major factor in aging, but it becomes a greater concern when blood glucose levels start to rise. Accelerated atherosclerosis, arthritis, dementia, skin wrinkling, leg ulcers, cataract formation and retinal eye damage found in diabetics is direct evidence of this process. Of further concern is the potential of "protein sticking" to disrupt immune function.

The end-products of protein-sticking are called "advanced glycation end products" (AGEs). From the concerns noted above to muscle weakness, accumulation of AGEs is a direct contributor to aging. AGE accumulation is, to some extent, unavoidable, but the process can be slowed by reducing carbohydrate intake. There's even some good news for individuals who have spent a lifetime overindulging on carbohydrates: the process is reversible! Reduction of carbohydrates to an acceptable level and high intake of vegetables allows mechanisms in the body to break down and remove AGEs.

◊*The degree of "protein sticking" (a process formally known as "glycation") can be detected easily by measuring the amount of glucose stuck to hemoglobin molecules (hemoglobin is the protein that carries oxygen in your blood). This test, called a Hemoglobin A1c, is useful for measuring the level of blood sugar control in a diabetic, but is also a useful measure of the degree of AGE's accumulation. The normal range is 3% to 6%. A diabetic with poor control may have values of 8 or greater and with good control, a value of about 6%. Most "normal" patients have levels of 5.5 to 6%, evidence of a very concerning trend in America. Less than 5.0% is the target level for optimal health.*

Most tissues of the body can use glucose for fuel, but the brain uses it almost exclusively. For this reason, the level of glucose in the bloodstream must be very tightly regulated. Too little, and the brain screams for more; too much, and the toxic effects of glucose quickly become apparent. This "glucose thermostat" is maintained by a complex series of hormones with the most important one being insulin.

When you take a bite out of a confection such as a donut, the starch and sugar are broken down into pure glucose almost before you taste the sweetness. The glucose is rapidly absorbed through the small intestine, sending a surge of glucose into your bloodstream that sets off alarm bells. In response, the hormone insulin (secreted by special cells in the pancreas) is immediately released. **Insulin sends a special message to the cells of your liver and muscle, allowing these tissues to take up the extra glucose, thus rapidly lowering your blood glucose back to normal.** Without insulin, this vital function cannot occur and blood glucose would continue to rise until you were quite ill.

A donut every now and then is okay, but eating a high starch and sugar diet on a daily basis can only lead to dire consequences. After being subjected to unremitting surges of glucose followed by compulsory surges in insulin, the cells of the liver and muscles finally say, "Enough is enough, and no more!" Like teenagers ignoring nagging parents, they just stop listening. The body cannot have this, of course, because high levels of glucose are toxic, so the pancreas is pushed to secrete ever higher amounts of insulin to force cells into accepting more glucose. The chronically elevated insulin levels that result create a vicious cycle that is referred to as *insulin resistance*. *Impaired glucose metabolism* is a more general term also used to describe the same process.

With time, worsening insulin resistance pushes the "glucose thermostat" ever upward, because higher levels of glucose are required to have the same effect. Insulin-producing cells in the pancreas gradually burn out and glucose levels rise even further—initially to a *pre-diabetic* level, but eventually to a level classified as *Type 2* diabetes, generally requiring medications or injections of insulin. The incidence of insulin resistance and Type 2 diabetes in this country is astoundingly high and still on the rise.

Basic screening for Type II diabetes can be done by measuring a simple "fasting blood glucose level." A value over 110 mg/dL is considered pre-diabetic, but anything over 100 mg/dL is a sign of diminishing pancreatic reserves. Overt diabetes is suspected with a value over 130 mg/dL.

For optimal health, fasting blood glucose should be maintained below 90 and hemoglobin A1c should be around 5.0 or below. Fasting blood glucose consistently >100 mg/dL suggests that the pancreas has lost half of its ability to produce insulin. This is a case where active therapy beyond dietary changes alone should be considered to compensate for cumulative damage.

Like most Americans, I consumed baked goods of various types throughout the day and with almost every meal. By age 45, I was fighting excessive weight continually, dealing with ravenous hunger and frequently experiencing episodes of hypoglycemia. Alarmed by fasting blood glucose of 110 and hemoglobin A1c of 5.9, I decided to get serious. I purchased a glucometer and starting checking my blood glucose levels—after fasting, two hours after meals and at random.

At first, virtually everything I ate shot my blood glucose into alarming ranges. Gradually, as I became savvy about food and types of carbohydrates, my blood glucose levels returned to within normal range and I was able to get control. My hemoglobin A1c is presently around 5.3 (Yes, I'm still working on it!).

To gain control, one the toughest things I gave up was wheat. Wheat products (white flour and whole grain alike, it didn't really matter) seemed to aggravate my blood glucose levels like nothing else. Once wheat was gone from my life, glucose control was less of a struggle and maintaining normal weight was easier. I felt remarkably better and my intestinal system began functioning properly for the first time ever. I have since made the same recommendation to countless individuals who have had the same response.

Not all of the sugar and starch in that donut are immediately burned for energy. The leftovers are stored for later use as *glycogen*, a substance similar to starch. Glycogen storage occurs in both liver and muscle tissue. This is very practical: when we go for periods without eating, glycogen can be readily converted back into glucose to bring blood levels back to normal. During intense exercise we depend on our glycogen stores, but they can become depleted. When runners talk about "hitting a wall," they have used up all of their glycogen.

Interestingly, chronically high insulin levels block the body's ability to break down glycogen. Without the ability to break down glycogen, blood glucose levels quickly crash if an insulin-resistant individual goes without eating or attempts vigorous exercise. In other words, if you live on a steady diet of processed carbohydrates, the body loses its ability to quickly compensate when blood glucose levels drop. This phenomenon, referred to as *hypoglycemia* (low blood sugar), translates into an insatiable hunger, craving for carbohydrates, and exercise intolerance. When you include the additional effect elevated insulin has of blocking fat from being removed from fat stores, chronic obesity is inevitable.

The feeling of shakiness and hunger commonly associated with hypoglycemia can occur at normal blood glucose levels in insulin-resistant individuals. As tissues become resistant to the effects of insulin, it takes higher levels of insulin and concomitantly higher levels of glucose to achieve the same result. The "glucose thermostat" is altered in an upward direction to maintain normalcy. A person with insulin resistance may start feeling uncomfortable at a blood glucose level of 90 or even as high as 100, and will need to maintain blood glucose in that range to feel comfortable. This translates into a higher level of tissue damage for the insulin-resistant individual, even though that person is not yet diabetic.

Any person with insulin resistance should be acutely aware of the fact that exercise allows glucose to enter cells without insulin. Regular exercise is one of the best ways to reverse the effects of insulin resistance and may help alter the set-point of the "glucose thermostat" in a positive way.

The transition from normal to type II diabetes is gradual and almost insidious. In the early stages of insulin resistance, fasting blood glucose may be perfectly normal. A person with fasting blood glucose of 83 could still be in the process of becoming insulin-resistant. As cells of the body become more resistant to insulin and the pancreas becomes more stressed, the "glucose thermostat" gradually rises toward a concerning level.

Formal testing for insulin resistance includes hourly measurements of glucose and insulin levels for three hours after consuming 100 grams of glucose (called a glucose tolerance test—3 hour GTT). But formal testing is

not always necessary; any person who displays a triad of weight gain, carbohydrate craving, and episodes of hypoglycemia while following an average American diet can be assumed to have impaired glucose metabolism, no matter what the lab values show.

The adverse effects of insulin resistance are not limited solely to weight gain and concern for diabetes. Chronically elevated insulin levels not only throw a monkey wrench into the entire glucose-regulating system, but also have a negative influence on all of the hormone systems of the body. This cascade of dysfunction impacts the adrenal hormones, the male and female reproductive hormones, and definitely affects the way the brain functions. Insulin and related insulin-like growth factors stimulate cell growth—a factor that many experts feel could play a role in inducing cancer.

The numbers of bake sales and doughnut drives going on to raise money for cancer research strongly suggests that the general public is not aware of the connection between insulin resistance and cancer. Even the academic community has not weighed in regarding this disservice. Physiologically, starchy treats actually promote conditions that may lead to certain cancers.

Elevated insulin levels and associated insulin-like growth factors promote cell growth and have been linked to initiation of cancer. Add to it the extra estrogen associated with increased abdominal fat and it is not surprising that postmenopausal obesity is one of the strongest predictors of breast cancer risk!

Once insulin resistance is established, it takes a while to reverse. Insulin-resistant individuals pursuing weight loss are often frustrated by this phenomenon—absolute reversal of the cellular changes associated with insulin resistance can take months. A better diet and regular exercise are a good place to start, but strict blood glucose control is essential. Many supplements and medications are available that can help the process.

Just shy of her twenty-fifth birthday, Irene presented to the office with complaints including irregular and sometimes heavy periods, weight gain across her middle abdomen, and acne. Other symptoms included carbohydrate craving and episodes of hypoglycemia. Her blood pressure was mildly elevated. Dietary history revealing high consumption of processed carbohydrates. She had been given a diagnosis of polycystic ovaries and was already on birth control pills to regulate her periods. Her mother was a nurse and had read that medications for diabetes could be helpful for treatment of polycystic ovaries. Surprisingly, however, her hemoglobin A1c was only 4.7, suggesting that she was far from being diabetic.

Often the diagnosis of insulin resistance remains elusive. Even though the hemoglobin A1c suggests that Irene's blood glucose levels have not started going up, all the signs point to insulin resistance as the root cause of her symptoms—as insulin resistance develops, insulin levels rise before glucose levels. Elevated insulin levels have adverse effects on not only adrenal hormones but also reproductive hormones. Female reproductive hormones are shifted toward a male pattern, causing acne and irregular periods. The change in adrenal hormones contributes to central obesity and hypertension. A high stress level adds fuel to the fire, throwing off adrenal hormones even further.

Irene was placed on a strict high vegetable, low-carb diet and a low dose anti-diabetic medication. She began working with a personal trainer several days a week and started exercising daily. At first it seemed her weight would never budge, but she did start feeling better almost immediately. Gradually the weight began to change and after a while, with her continued persistence, it fell off precipitously. Eventually she was able to stop the medication and all of her symptoms resolved.

THE CHOLESTEROL CONNECTION

Like so many individuals, for many years I carried the belief that cholesterol problems arose from consuming too much meat, eggs and dairy. Though diets high in saturated fat also tend to also be high in cholesterol, dietary cholesterol, except in rare incidences, is not the source of high blood cholesterol. Only 25% of cholesterol in the body comes from dietary sources; the remaining 75% is synthesized by the liver. Problems with cholesterol stem from the body's incessant ability to manufacture cholesterol and gradual loss of the ability to properly get rid of it!

It seems counterintuitive, but problems with elevated cholesterol are more related to consuming a low fiber, high glucose diet than to eating too much fat! Here's why: By the third donut of the morning your glycogen stores are completely topped off for the day and not much energy is required for sitting at a desk. The extra glucose building up in your bloodstream has to go somewhere. That somewhere is the adipose tissue around your middle. Conversion of glucose to fat occurs primarily in the liver. **Newly formed fat must be transported from its origins in the liver to the adipose tissue of the body via the bloodstream.**

This presents a problem. As you know, fat and water do not mix very well. To solve this dilemma, the liver is able to synthesize special particles called *lipoproteins.* Lipoproteins consist of a microscopic globule of fat enveloped with a layer of protein, allowing the particle to be soluble in the blood. Cholesterol is a necessary add-on to keep the particle stable and is therefore an essential ingredient for the creation of lipoprotein particles.

Although cholesterol carries a negative image in many peoples' minds, it is vital for many functions within the human body. Not only does it stabilize lipoprotein particles, but it also stabilizes all of the cell membranes in the body. Cholesterol is the precursor for many hormones in the body and is an essential component of bile, necessary for the digestion of fat. The body considers cholesterol to be a precious substance and carefully re-circulates it. As we could never depend on dietary sources alone to provide all that we need, the body has a significant capacity to not only manufacture it, but also to conserve it. In fact, cholesterol inside the body only becomes a problem when it is not properly re-circulated.

A newly formed lipoprotein particle travels from the liver to adipose tissue via the bloodstream. On arrival at the adipose tissue, the fatty contents of the particle are disgorged into a fat cell. The leftover particle, now containing mainly cholesterol and protein, is left floating around in the bloodstream. **This particle, referred to as LDL (low density lipo-protein), is the one your doctor is worried about.**

Much of the cholesterol found in LDL particles does end up back in the cholesterol re-circulation pathway, but not all of it. The liver acts like a net that captures vagrant LDL particles as they pass through the bloodstream. LDL particles, however, vary in size. Smaller particles tend to slip through the net and remain floating in the bloodstream, thus remaining a threat. Fortunately all is not lost, as a scavenger particle, called HDL, picks up cholesterol and adds it to smaller LDL particles, such that they can be "caught" by the liver and re-circulated. HDL particles are the good guys. **Risk of atherosclerosis is partially defined by the amounts of HDL particles as compared to small LDL particles.**

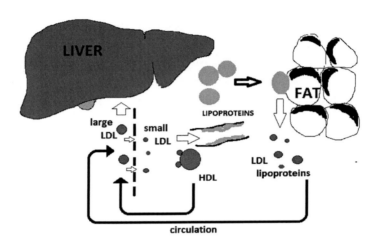

Type II diabetes is typically associated with low levels of HDL and abnormally high concentrations of small particle LDL. Elevated insulin and high carbohydrate intake induce increased amounts of free fats called triglycerides in the blood. This triad—low HDL, small particle LDL, and elevated triglycerides—is commonly found in steady consumers of grain-source carbohydrates (especially wheat). These people may not yet be diabetic, but are usually on their way to becoming impaired. Substitute high quantities of vegetables, reduce grain consumption and the pattern typically shifts to a favorable ratio—with no drugs required!

THE SILENT THREAT OF ATHEROSCLEROSIS

Though risk is often linked primarily to LDL cholesterol levels, cardiovascular disease is, more than anything else, a flow problem. Compromised blood flow to vital organs is devastating. If blood were as thin as water, flow would not be a problem, but blood is viscous. The increased viscosity of blood is related to all the stuff in it. Even though blood acts like a liquid, it contains solid, partially dissolved and dissolved components including red blood cells, white blood cells, proteins, fat (triglycerides), lipoprotein particles, nutrients, immune factors, platelets and coagulation factors—whew! That's a complex mix! A significant force must be generated by heart to push it through blood vessels.

The Cattleman's Beef Board has correctly pointed out the beef does not raise cholesterol. The saturated fat in beef does, however, increase viscosity, and therefore risk.

Viscous blood flowing through blood vessels creates friction. Friction causes damage to the lining of vessels. Blood vessels where flow and turbulence are high, such as arteries supplying the brain and heart, are most affected. Increased viscosity equates with increased friction and therefore increased damage. Like a scab that forms on scraped skin, the body tries to heal the injury. Coagulation factors including fibrin and platelets are laid down on the injured surface and white blood cells are called in for repair. In this case, however, the healing process increases friction and a vicious cycle is created.

Stress, usually a part of a high-risk lifestyle, increases platelet "stickiness." (Of course, while running from a tiger, you would want your blood to clot easily in case you became slashed!)

The lesion that forms is referred to as plaque. Vagrant LDL particles become embedded in the mix and accelerate plaque formation. Small LDL particles that have been "oxidized" by free radicals are the most problematic. Free radicals, as we know, are chemical substances that have the potential to do damage to living tissue. Free radicals that accelerate plaque formation come from different sources. Toxins in cigarette smoke would be a good example. Abnormal fats found in processed and fried foods are notorious for increasing the presence of free radicals in the bloodstream. Free radicals can also be produced by the inflammatory cells of the immune system as part of our defense mechanisms. Any inflammatory process can contribute to the problem; chronic sinusitis, arthritis, inflammatory bowel disease and even periodontal (gum) disease, can be associated with an increased risk of cardiovascular disease.

Though microbes are not commonly implicated in the process of atherosclerosis, the association between periodontal disease and cardiovascular disease would suggest a link. In fact, evidence of pathogenic bacteria commonly causing gum disease has been found within arterial plaques. These bacteria reside in "biofilms" which are shielded by gelatinous coats that are highly resistant to antibiotic penetration. Possibly not by coincidence alone, early arterial plaques resemble the structure of a biofilm. (Circulation, volume 113(7) p. 920-922, Katz and Shannon)

The process of atherosclerosis, as described above, is a major cause of premature morbidity and mortality in this country. As we age we must become increasingly vigilant about reducing the threat of atherosclerosis. A comprehensive approach should go well beyond simply lowering cholesterol. Risk reduction should include a strategy to reduce blood viscosity and improve blood flow. A healthy diet, regular exercise and stress reduction address all factors associated with risk. Risk reduction can be accentuated with properly chosen natural supplements. Pharmaceutical therapy is sometimes necessary to adequately control cardiovascular risk, but drug therapy should always be used in conjunction with natural therapy and used at the lowest possible doses.

TAKE HEART! Atherosclerosis is reversible! Atherosclerotic plaques will shrink with proper dietary changes, exercise, stress reduction, appropriate supplements and medications[*]. See www.vitalplan.com, RESTORE, Cardiovascular Health, for more information.

---

[*] Risk of atherosclerosis in conventional medicine today is addressed almost exclusively by lowering cholesterol with medications called statins. While there is a place for these medications, their use is associated with significant side effects, including skeletal muscle pain, depletion of certain nutrients and increased risk of heart failure secondary to compromise of heart muscle function.

◊Most healthcare providers order a lipid panel, where cholesterol is broken down into different lipoprotein particles. Ever wondered what those numbers mean? Total cholesterol is less important than the values of the subcomponents. LDL cholesterol, the most concerning particles, should ideally have a value below 130 mg/dL. A normal HDL value is above 40, but the higher the better; values above 60 are more ideal. Risk of atherosclerosis is best evaluated by looking at the ratio between LDL and HDL. Ideally, the LDL/HDL ratio should be less than 4.5. For optimal health, the ratio should be less than 3.5. Supplements and sometimes carefully-chosen medications can be beneficial for achieving this goal.

One step better is measuring particle size of both LDL and HDL particles. Smaller particles of both HDL and LDL translate into higher risk.

Complete risk assessment includes measurement of C-reactive protein, an indicator of inflammation (and oxidative stress) in the bloodstream. For optimal health, the C-reactive protein level should be less than 1.0.

FRUCTOSE: THE OTHER SIMPLE CARBOHYDRATE

Fructose, commonly known as fruit sugar, is the darling of the commercial food industry. Sweeter than table sugar and less expensive to produce, it is almost ubiquitous in processed foods and drinks. The addictive nature of the sweetness alone makes it an attractive addition to products, but fructose holds another ace—it actually disrupts hunger control mechanisms. Whereas consumption of glucose activates hormones that *suppress* appetite, fructose actually blocks these hormones and thus encourages overeating. After one "super-size-me" fructose-filled soft drink, it's almost impossible not to go back for another helping of food!

This fact alone should be reason enough to seriously monitor fructose consumption, but health concerns do not stop here. Fructose has a much higher affinity for proteins than glucose, compounding the "protein-sticking" effect on aging and disease. Fructose, converted to fat, increases cardiovascular risk and metabolism of fructose increases uric acid, contributing elevated blood pressure and gout. Insulin has no effect on fructose, therefore blood levels are not tightly regulated and the potential for damage increases with amounts consumed.

Natural concentrations of fructose found in fruit can be a concern with over-consumption, but artificially high concentrations of fructose introduced into processed foods and beverages are the real problem. High-fructose corn syrup historically has been the primary offender, but as the general public becomes more "health" conscious, the commercial food industry is shifting to fructose in a different form—concentrated fructose-laden "natural" fruit juices—to sweeten foods.

THE DISACCHARIDES

Sucrose: Ordinary table sugar, from sugar cane or sugar beets, is actually a "double sugar" made from a molecule of glucose bonded to a molecule of fructose. Enzymes in the intestine free the bond, releasing equal amounts of glucose and fructose. An occasional teaspoon of sugar to sweeten coffee or tea can brighten the day, but the mountains of sugar consumed by Americans each year is clearly over the top.

Lactose: Commonly known as "milk sugar," lactose is also a double sugar comprised of a molecule of glucose and a molecule of a sugar called galactose. Many adults lack the enzyme lactase, which is necessary to break down milk products. Without this enzyme, undigested lactose flushes through the intestinal tract, causing diarrhea and flatulence. Lactose-intolerant individuals should generally avoid all milk products with the exception of fermented products such as yogurt. Even for lactose-tolerant individuals, excessive consumption contributes to glucose impairment and galactose has some of the same problems as fructose.

FAT

From a dietary point of view, fats are just as important as sugars for maintaining normal health. These molecules come in many different shapes and sizes, and they have numerous functions within the human body. In the case of dietary fats, the *type* of fat is as important as the *amount* of fat. While the right fats can add to your health in many ways, the wrong fats can make you very ill.

MISCONCEPTIONS ABOUT FAT

Beyond excessive carbohydrates, processed food diets are notorious for being fat offenders. Cheeseburgers, hotdogs, fried chicken and sausage biscuits are, of course, laden with fat, but health concerns goes beyond their contribution to obesity alone. The potential for harm associated with dietary fat is directly related to processing before consumption.

Fat plays a much larger role in the body than just providing an energy source. Many normal functions within the human body involve fats; the inventory of fats influences how well these functions will occur. The three main categories of fat to know about include saturated fat, polyunsaturated fat and mono-unsaturated fat. Each category of fat comes in many forms, and different forms serve different purposes within the body.

The chemical structure of a saturated fat is that of a long straight chain. Different saturated fats come in different lengths (long-chain, medium-chain and short-chain). Saturated fats tend to stack closely together and are therefore solid at room temperature. The fatty chains found in polyunsaturated fats contain several chemical links called double-bonds that "kink" the chain at these locations. These bent fat chains do not stack well and are therefore exist as liquid at room temperature. The double bonds, however, make polyunsaturated fats very susceptible to damage by free radicals. Monounsaturated fats have only one double bond in the chain and are therefore less susceptible to free-radical damage. Though they have only one double bond, they are kinked enough to be liquid at room temperature. These fats are generally healthful. Olive oil is an example of a monounsaturated fat.

There is no doubt that baked goods plump up better and taste better when made with saturated fat. Your great-grandmother always used lard or butter to make biscuits, but biscuits may not have been an everyday affair because animal fats were expensive and did not keep well. A new age of cooking was ushered in when the Crisco Company introduced vegetable shortening in 1911. For a fraction of the cost of animal fat, liquid poly-unsaturated vegetable oil could be made into saturated fat by a process known as "hydrogenation." Margarine is made by this same process. Though margarine and vegetable shortening may look and taste very similar to their animal source equivalents, hydrogenation causes unnatural changes to the oil, leaving it of questionable value for human consumption.

If all of the fat we consumed each day was immediately burned, the source and type would actually not matter very much, but the role of fat in the human body goes well beyond energy production. The old saying, "you are what you eat" is very accurate when it comes to fat. All of the trillions of cells in our bodies are individually surrounded by a membrane that is composed of a double layer of specialized fat. Altogether, this adds up to a significant amount of fat. Most of the lipids (fats) within your cell membranes come from fat that is consumed. **In fact, any type of fat that is consumed has the potential to end up in your cell membranes!**

CELL MEMBRANE STRUCTURE

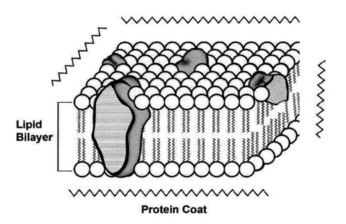

Cell membranes deserve more attention than they get. Everything that the cell needs to function must come through the membrane. Some substances diffuse directly through the membrane and others are transported across by specialized proteins floating within the membrane. Other types of specialized proteins within the membrane act as receptors for hormones or other chemical messengers that direct functions within the cell. In short, cell membranes are vital for normal function of every cell within the body. If your cell membranes are not up to par, you cannot expect to feel well.

A diet high in *saturated fat* or *hydrogenated fat* creates cell membranes that are stiff (think lard or vegetable shortening). From a functional point of view, this is not how you want your cell membranes to be. Liquid fat (oil) makes the membrane more fluid, and therefore more functional, but there is a tradeoff. Excessive amounts of poly-unsaturated fats make cell membranes very susceptible to damage by free radicals. **Refined oils and hydrogenated oils contain fats that have already become free radicals and are therefore extremely damaging to cell membranes!**

"Trans-fats," that you hear so much about, are polyunsaturated fats that have been shifted into unnatural configurations by high heat or chemicals. This abnormal configuration does not mesh well with other, normal lipids in the cell membrane and can disrupt membrane function. You really do not want trans-fats cluttering up your cell membranes!

Deep frying, a central component of the American fast food scene, requires hot, liquid oil. The least expensive oils are derived from vegetable sources, most commonly corn or soybean. Vegetable oil consists mainly of poly-unsaturated fat. Poly-unsaturated fats are very fragile and susceptible to damage by heat. Inexpensive vegetable oils are "refined" or extracted from the original source using high heat and harsh chemicals. This process damages the fat and creates abnormal fats that act as free radicals and become the infamous "trans-fats" that everyone is worried about. Pour this oil into a large vat and heat it to the temperature required for deep fat frying, and you have a real caldron of toxic substances on your hands.

Recently I was amused to read that several states have banned the use of trans-fats for deep fat frying in restaurants. Tran- fats do not occur readily in nature and are not present in vegetable oil before it is extracted from the plant. Tran- fats are created when the poly-unsaturated fat (oil) extracted from a plant such as corn is exposed to high heat during the extraction process. Exposure to high heat associated with deep fat frying actually creates trans-fats. Even if you start with "trans-fat- free" oil, trans-fats will be created during the deep fat frying process. Sometimes we do the most nonsensical things.

Mono-unsaturated fats are the types of fat that you do want to have in your cell membranes. These fats, commonly found in olive oil, nuts and avocados, increase resistance to oxidation, maintain membrane fluidity and allow optimal cell membrane function. Possibly the healthiest cell membranes are those composed predominantly of mono-saturated fat with just a little touch of saturated fat thrown in for good measure.

In limited amounts, saturated fat is not all bad. It is extremely stable and resistant to damage by free radicals. This is a very desirable quality and having just the right amount of it in cell membranes is valuable. Though saturated fat, layered into an established plaque, contributes to the process of cardiovascular disease, it is usually not the primary inciting factor.

Fat, in general, is absorbed directly through the intestines and is transported through the bloodstream to other parts of the body via a different system of lipoproteins than used for glucose-derived fat. Though excessive consumption of saturated fat can contribute to the process of plaque formation, excessive *carbohydrate* consumption seems to be a greater contributor. In actuality, the health concern associated with consumption of saturated fat in foods such as beef, pork, and dairy products has as much to do with toxins dissolved in the fat and imbalances in a special group of fats called "essential fatty acids" than it has to do with the saturated fat itself.

Essential fatty acids (EFA's) are a special group of polyunsaturated fats termed "essential" because they cannot be synthesized by the body and must be obtained from dietary sources. Getting enough EFA's to survive is generally not a problem because they are abundant in the foods we eat, but getting the right ratio of the right types is a different story altogether. Essential fatty acids have many important functions in the human body, from contributing to healthy cell membranes to regulation of inflammation in the body.

The process of inflammation is intended to be part of a healing process. Our immune system is constantly correcting damage caused by free radicals, toxins, invading microbes and the like. This very complex system requires careful orchestration of specialized cells found in the bloodstream and other parts of the body. Various types of chemical messengers are used to organize an inflammatory response. Many of these chemical messengers are derived from essential fatty acids. A correct balance of different types of EFA's is important: With just the right balance of essential fatty acids, health is optimized; however, too much of one type of essential fatty acid may lead to an exaggerated inflammatory response commonly known as inflammation.

The types and amounts of essential fatty acids that we consume very much influence the inflammatory response in our bodies. The average American diet is very high in the essential fatty acids termed *Omega-6* but very low in *Omega-3*. Certain types of Omega-6 EFA's tend to heighten the inflammatory response while Omega-3 EFA's tend to moderate it. So, in terms of essential fatty acids, average American diets are very "pro-inflammatory." Grain-fed livestock and poultry are high in inflammation-inducing Omega-6 and very low in Omega-3. The opposite would be preferred (for the animal and for us). When these same animals are allowed to eat natural grasses (i.e. free-range) they have much higher levels of Omega-3's. Oily fish such as mackerel, tuna, salmon and sardines are naturally high in these important essential fatty acids. Vegetarian sources of omega-3's include algae, flax seed oil, borage oil, and walnuts.

◊*The ratio of omega-6 to omega-3 fatty acids can be measured. For optimal health, the ratio for reduced inflammatory response is 4:1. The average ratio for most Americans is closer to 20:1 or even 30:1. When omega-3 saturation testing becomes standardized, it may develop into an optimal test for predicting the incidence of both atherosclerosis and chronic disease.*

Omega-3 EFA's have other benefits, too: for example, they help to prevent oxidation of "LDL" cholesterol. This may be more important in preventing arterial plaque formation than lowering the cholesterol. In addition, EFA's act as a mild blood thinner, essential for protecting arteries against plaque formation. Diets higher in Omega-3 EFA's tend to lower one's risk of inflammatory diseases such as arthritis and atherosclerosis, and likely also decrease risks of cancer. **A high-quality "fish oil" or essential fatty acid supplement is the one dietary supplement that everyone over the age of 40 should consider.**

PROTEINS

Proteins are responsible for a wide range of functions within the human body. They are, in essence, what makes us tick. Thousands of different types of proteins perform a mind-boggling number of functions within the human body.

These vital proteins include the following:
- *Enzymes, responsible for regulating all of the biochemical reactions necessary for life, are proteins. Often these enzymes require vital cofactors in the form of vitamins and minerals to function properly.*

- *Specialized proteins allow muscles to contract, skin to stretch, and hormones to work.*

- *Found in our blood, the hemoglobin molecule carries oxygen; other blood proteins are responsible for carrying nutrients and hormones throughout the body and also act as buffers to regulate blood pH.*

- *Antibodies and some other essential parts of the immune system are proteins that protect us from foreign invaders.*

- *Proteins are an integral part of all cell membranes. Some regulate the passage of substances in and out of the cell; other cell membrane proteins are receptors for chemical messengers.*

The most basic components of proteins are molecules called amino acids. There are about twenty amino acids used to make proteins in the body, but many other amino acids occur in nature. Nine amino acids are considered "essential," meaning they cannot be synthesized by the body and must be obtained from dietary sources.

One of the primary uses of amino acids is in protein synthesis. Long chains of amino acids are linked together to form the basic protein structure. The chain is then folded several times to create the final protein. The exact sequences of amino acids are coded for by DNA within our genes. **Mutations in our genes can mean improper coding which results in formation of abnormal proteins.**

Amino acids can be linked to form shorter chains called peptides. Many of our hormones are peptides or polypeptides. Insulin is a good example of a polypeptide hormone. The sequence of the amino acids determines the function of the polypeptide.

Amino acids have other vital functions besides the formation of peptide chains and proteins. Amino acids themselves can be chemical messengers or can be modified into other chemical messengers within the body. Some of these amino acids are not ever found in proteins. The neurotransmitters epinephrine, dopamine, GABA and serotonin found within the nervous system and brain are examples of chemical messengers made from amino acids. Thyroid hormones are modified amino acids. Certain amino acids are even precursors to the molecules that make up our DNA.

Another important function of amino acids is protection from free-radicals. Several amino acids containing sulfur groups can be converted into a chemical called *glutathione*. Glutathione is present in all cells and is a remarkably important antioxidant. *Glutathione* is especially important in liver cells where detoxification occurs. Adequate sources of these amino acids are necessary for glutathione synthesis. Also, Vitamin C and vitamin E are essential for regeneration of glutathione.

Proteins in the body continuously wear out and need to be replaced. Worn-out proteins are broken down into component amino acids, which are often reused. Protein, lost from the body via metabolism, urine, feces, and menstrual flow contributes to the constant turnover. Amino acids are also lost via metabolism for energy production or conversion into other vital chemicals. Our bodies use about 80 to 100 grams of protein each day. A moderate dietary intake of protein is necessary to replace daily protein and amino acid losses. Fortunately, in America, sources of quality dietary protein are readily available.

The quality of dietary protein is assessed by the assortment of amino acids contained. A complete protein source offers all of the essential amino acids. If a single essential amino acid is regularly missing from the diet, protein synthesis may be hampered.

Eggs are often the standard by which all other dietary proteins are graded. Eggs are considered a complete source of protein as they contain all of the necessary amino acids for protein synthesis including all of the essential amino acids. Eggs also contain vital minerals and many important chemicals substances. Other complete sources of protein include dairy products, meat, fish, and shellfish and soybeans. Adequate dietary protein can easily be obtained from vegetarian sources by combining foods. Certain plants may not be complete protein sources in themselves, but they may contain essential amino acids that others do not have. Varying foods such as brown rice with wheat, nuts, beans, or other seeds provides a complete source of protein.

The body has the ability to break down proteins to use as a primary energy source but only elects to do so in a pinch. It would be analogous to pealing the planks off a wooden ship to burn them in the engine room. Proteins from food sources, broken down into component amino acids in the intestines, can also be used as an energy source, but they are best used to make new proteins. Amino acids only become a primary energy source in the absence of sugars.[*] The body must actually expend more energy to use amino acids as an energy source. This is the premise behind weight loss using low-carbohydrate diets.

If by this point you have decided to exclude <u>all</u> dietary carbohydrates and join the throngs of people who have turned to strictly low-carb, high protein, high fat diets, you should think twice. Without carbohydrates, fat and protein become the primary energy sources for the body. Fat is good for the "slow burn" but is a poor source of quick energy needed for activities such as thinking or sprinting. Amino acids can be used for quick energy, but are not designed to do so—they do not work as well and their leftover by-products are toxic. "Brain fog," arthritis, gout, immune suppression and loss of calcium from bones are just a few of the concerns associated with high protein diets.

Another variation on the theme is the "Paleo diet." While we can and should learn from what our long-gone ancestors typically ate, the fact that the average primitive man was lucky to reach age 35 adds little credibility to the diet. A better example of how to live and eat would be offered by studying the people on the island of Okinawa, Japan. Islanders following traditional diets routinely live past 80 and frequently reach 100! While their diet is very high in vegetables, it does include soy, meat, and carbohydrates from grain and fruit sources. Their omega-6 to omega-3 ratio is the ideal 4:1!

---

[*] The intestines do use certain amino acids as a primary fuel source, but this is a minor part of the total energy consumption of the body.

As with many things, the answer is moderation. Healthy sources of fats, proteins __and__ carbohydrates are part and parcel of a healthful diet. High vegetable intake is the key to making it healthy. The high fiber and phytonutrients found in vegetables slow absorption of glucose from grains and other sources, remove toxins and reduces cholesterol, improve gastrointestinal function and allow proper assimilation of other nutrients.

VITAMINS AND MINERALS

Vitamins are chemical substances that must be obtained from dietary sources. Without these vital chemicals, key reactions in the body would not occur and life would not be possible. The classic vitamins include A, B, C, D, E, and K. While knowing all the details of each vitamin is not necessary, it is important to note that the letters represent "families" of chemicals and not just one single chemical. There are many different types of B vitamins and vitamin E comes in at least eight different forms (a fact that seems to be lost on many vitamin supplement manufacturers who supply only one synthetic form of each vitamin in their "once-a-days").

It is also important to note that the different vitamins are not related chemicals. Being distinctly different, they come from different food sources. This is one of the reasons why it is so vital to eat a wide variety of foods. All of the vitamins, with the exception of one, can be obtained from plant sources. Vitamin B-12 is synthesized only by bacteria and is acquired only by consuming meat products or through supplements.

Besides vitamins, there are many other key chemicals required for the body's vital reactions. These chemical substances differ from the classic vitamins in that the body has the ability to synthesize them; dietary sources are not essential. Even so, acquiring these substances from food sources saves the body work and energy—another good reason to follow a healthy diet. As we age, our bodies gradually lose the ability to produce some of these substances. Co-enzyme Q-10, a key chemical necessary for energy production, is one example. Some people over fifty will experience less daily fatigue when taking a co-enzyme Q-10 supplement.

A commonly asked question is why some vital substances can be synthesized by the body and others, termed essential, must be obtained from dietary sources. The answer probably has to do with availability of foods as humans evolved. Very likely, substances that we now call vitamins were so readily available from dietary sources that certain organisms simply gave up the ability to make them—why waste energy on something that is already there? A good example is vitamin C. Humans and other primates are the only higher animals that cannot synthesize vitamin C, evidence suggesting that the diets of primitive humans were very high in vitamin C.

Minerals from the earth are vital for all living organisms. Bones would not be possible without calcium and phosphorus. Our hemoglobin could not carry oxygen without iron. Thyroid hormones depend on iodine. Fluctuations in sodium and potassium ions are essential for many cellular functions. The immune system depends on both zinc and selenium. All the minerals required by the body for daily functions must be obtained from dietary sources and are readily present in a varied diet of whole foods.

Minerals are important for maintaining normal pH in the bloodstream and tissues of the body. Optimal pH for all chemical functions in the body is 7.4. Slightly alkaline pH keeps calcium and other minerals in bones and is associated with good health in general. The best way to maintain slightly alkaline pH is by regularly consuming vegetables and fruit. The regular dietary addition of unrefined sea salt may also help to maintain a slightly alkaline pH.

Processed foods, refined sugar, soft drinks and high protein diets push the body toward acidic pH. Beyond being associated with poor health in general, this may be a significant contributing factor to early loss of bone density and osteoporosis, which is now at near epidemic levels in the United States.

Though some minerals naturally found in the soil are beneficial for living organisms, others are actually poisonous. Metals including mercury, cadmium, aluminum, beryllium, lead and arsenic are quite toxic. These substances are not found to significant degree in natural foods and are by-products of industrialization and industrial food production. A healthy diet not only reduces exposure, but also helps the body rid itself of these toxic substances.

PHYTO-NUTRIENTS

Plants contain thousands of different types of chemical compounds that are commonly referred to as "phytochemicals." These chemical compounds are the ingredients that give a vegetable or fruit its distinct flavor; a factor that steers many people toward concoctions of fat and sugar which provide an intense taste of sweet, but offer little actual flavor. Anyone, however, can and should learn to enjoy these flavors, because they are important keys to enjoying a disease-free life.

Phytochemicals have many disease and cancer fighting attributes. Cruciferous vegetables (cabbage, broccoli, Brussels sprouts, cauliflower, kale are common examples) have been associated with diseases-fighting qualities since the beginning of recorded history and recently have been linked to reducing estrogen-related cancers. Berries contain chemicals with antioxidant, anti-inflammatory, anti-microbial and anti-cancer properties. Natural chemicals found in artichoke are potent antioxidants, lower cholesterol and at the same time, protect liver function. An unassuming stalk of celery offers potent cancer-inhibiting chemicals, lowers blood pressure in hypertensive individuals, is a mild sedative and raises testosterone levels in men. Green tea, soy and tomatoes are other important anti-cancer foods. All culinary spices have medicinal value. Turmeric (found in curries) and ginger are known for potent anti-inflammatory properties. Both also have important cancer-preventing properties. Garlic and onions contribute to reducing many types of disease.

These are just a few important examples. Virtually all fruits and vegetables offer some disease-fighting value. The disease-fighting capacity of a donut? Less than zero.

See Appendix B for information about nutritional supplements.

DIETARY FIBER

Dietary fiber includes all of the indigestible material in our food. Most of it comes from plant carbohydrates. Soluble fiber is made up of indigestible material that dissolves in water. Insoluble fiber makes up the bulk of stool and is not soluble in water. Both soluble and insoluble fiber are essential for normal health. Normal bowel function does not occur without adequate fiber. Fiber also aids in removal of toxins and excessive cholesterol, and it slows the absorption of glucose, helping to avoid insulin spikes. Though dietary fiber is not a source of energy or nutrients for us, certain types of fiber are a source of energy and nutrients for favorable bacteria in the large colon.

For optimal function, the waste disposal and detoxification systems of the body require a minimum of about 25 grams of dietary fiber every day. (An average American diet contains only about 5 to 10 grams.) Adequate dietary fiber, both soluble and insoluble, can easily be obtained by consuming a variety of vegetables, fruit, and to a lesser extent, whole grains.

Just the right amount of dietary glucose and other sugars found in whole foods are essential for good health. Healthy fats are essential to balance the cell membranes of the body. Adequate dietary protein must be present to offset daily turnover. Normal gastrointestinal function depends on fiber and vital chemical reactions would not occur without vital chemicals and minerals. Vegetables and fruits provide a host of disease-fighting phytochemicals. Mother Nature supplies the "right amounts" of each of these components in a well-proportioned diet made up of a variety of fresh, whole foods.

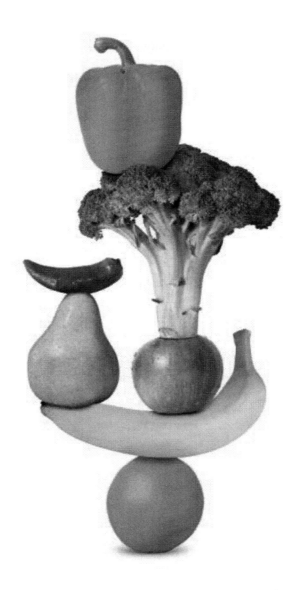

CHAPTER 7

Getting to Know Your Food

Imagine an island.

With a moderate climate, the most likely location of the island would be in the Mediterranean or possibly off of New Zealand. The terrain of the island is mountainous in the central region with rolling hills and fertile valleys near the coast. Because of the central mountain range, the island is very wet on the side exposed to trade winds and dry on the opposite side. The air and water are fresh and clean. The growing season is long and a wide variety of fruits and vegetables can be produced year round. Coffee, tea, and cool weather crops are grown in the mountains. Vineyards and several wineries are located on the dry side. Olive trees grow locally and olive oil is a staple. Coconut trees are, of course, found along the beaches.

Small farms provide fresh eggs and unrefined dairy products. They also provide chicken, pork, and lamb in limited quantities. Beef is available, but rare. Seafood of all kinds is plentiful from the clean waters that surround the island. Fresh food is distributed at open-air markets found at several locations. At the markets you will also find fresh nuts, spices and fresh herbs. Small local groceries provide bulk goods such as basmati rice, beans and pre-industrial-age grains. A stone mill will grind the grain into coarse flour for you to bake bread yourself, or you might patronize a bakery in the center of town that makes fresh whole grain breads daily. When planning a trip to the market, don't forget to bring your own containers, because nothing is encased in plastic.

Something to notice about the island is the absence of large grocery store chains. Processed and packaged foods, so common in America grocery stores, are too expensive to ship to the island and would go stale by the time they were sold. The islanders prefer food prepared fresh. Even the local restaurants and cafes prepare everything from scratch. Do not plan on fast food for lunch, as the midday meal is something to be savored.

I would have fared well being raised on such an island, but as it was, I grew up in the middle of the fast-food generation. For the longest time I thought Jimmy Buffet wrote "Cheeseburgers in Paradise" just for me—preferably two, with a whole plate of fries on the side. For most of my youth, I bought into the concept of fast food—hook, line, and sinker. And why not? Everything tasted good, didn't take any effort, and was available anytime you wanted it. Instant food, instant gratification. All that was necessary was a trip through the drive-thru, and a hot meal at home was as simple as browning a pound of hamburger and emptying the contents of a box into a skillet. Food was simple. Life was good.

As I crept into my thirties an expanding midline informed me that things were changing. Concern for a better diet was gradually forcing itself into my conscious thinking, but life was busy and change does not come easily. By mid-forties my blood pressure was creeping up a bit along with my blood glucose. A mid-morning snack and another one mid-afternoon had become a necessity to circumvent bouts of low blood sugar. This was occurring despite of the fact that I had become more nutritionally aware. My dietary habits had improved significantly, except for a cake and cookie addiction that I just could not shake. Starches and sugar had to go, but I was having a heck of a time giving them up.

Living on that island devoid of poor food choices would make switching to a healthier diet much easier, but life is never quite so simple. Finding healthier foods is not half as difficult as finding ways to incorporate them into daily life.

All of the healthy food choices available on the island can be readily found almost anywhere in America, but giving up all the unhealthy stuff is quite a challenge!

The first stage of my personal epicurean evolution included foods that *appeared* to be healthier versions of those to which I was already accustomed. Whole grains seemed to be a better choice, but my diet still consisted mainly of "healthier" forms of processed food. I call this my "granola bar and soy-burger phase." In an effort to be "totally healthy" I was not eating very much meat and was almost a vegetarian, though in retrospect my daily consumption of fresh vegetables was rather limited. This diet phase still contained a fair amount of "hidden" glucose and was heavy on grains. Because of their fat content I avoided foods that I now recognize as being healthy, such as nuts, eggs, and seafood. Gradually my nutritional education matured. Years of searching through both technical and non-technical information about nutrition all boiled down to basic common sense:

Healthy food, whether from vegetable or animal sources, is food that is closer to its natural origins.

Healthy food always starts with healthy soil. Topsoil, in its natural state, is a dynamic mixture of sand, clay, water and organic matter. It is very much alive with a complex assortment of organisms including thousands of different types of bacteria, fungi, protozoa, insects and worms. Though these lowly creatures do not sound very important, they are vital to the decomposition of dead plants and animals, providing nutrients for new plant growth. This is an essential cycle of life. Any organic farmer will tell you this is the optimal way to provide nutrients for a healthy plant. Beyond the absence of toxic chemicals, organically grown food from living soil is much higher in nutrients that are important for our health.

Unfortunately, the vast majority of our food is *not* produced in living soil. Excessive tillage and pesticide use in modern agriculture destroys the living organisms within the soil. Without the natural decomposition of organic matter, a substantial amount of nutrients have to be artificially added back in the form of fertilizer. Mother

Nature is hard to duplicate, and fertilizer never matches the nutrient capacity and delivery of dynamic, living soil. The practice of growing monocultures of the same crops year after year depletes the soil even further. Raw food materials are then processed, pasteurized, homogenized, and pulverized into the nutritionally deficient commercial food products found on most grocery store shelves. As if this were not enough, extensive hybridization and genetic engineering have changed the actual composition of many foods.

As I understood more about food, I realized my approach to food was going to have to change. It just did not make sense to regularly consume food that was obviously unhealthy, no matter how good it tasted. I decided that my shopping cart would no longer contain food items made with wheat flour, high fructose corn syrup and hydrogenated oil. I would not be visiting most of the aisles in the grocery store. Donuts and cakes I encountered daily would just have to go stale or be eaten by some other unfortunate soul. I would not be stopping at convenience marts or hording packaged snack foods to ward off bouts of low blood sugar. Fast food would be off-limits except for dire emergencies. *I would abstain.*

Compromises in life are often necessary. Food was going to cost a bit more, and I might have to make more effort to find quality food. Food products would have to be scrutinized carefully before being placed in the shopping cart. I would have to get to know the farmer down the road and search out local markets and vegetable stands. I might want to till a garden. Cooking more frequently would be a necessity. Tastes would have to change.

As with any change, changing to a better diet did not come easily, but change came with an almost unexpected transformation over a relatively short period of time. I immediately felt better. My taste buds gradually came alive as though they had been in a deep sleep. The sugar craving and episodes of hypoglycemia gradually subsided. My weight dropped! With time the new foods that at first tasted a bit odd became everyday staples and the processed stuff that I left behind began to seem as palatable as Play-dough. A whole world of new foods opened up before my eyes. Healthy foods, combined with just the right amount of sugar, fat, and spices showed the potential of being quite appealing. An almost unlimited number of flavor sensations were possible.

Healthy food gradually became synonymous with tasty food!

I have since come to think of my food only as "real" food—an apple as an apple. I do not want to know my food as a collection of processed flour, hydrogenated oil, high fructose corn syrup, polysorbate 80, red dye #53, and seasonings. What are those extras, anyway? The only label I want to see on my apple is one that defines where it came from and whether it is organic or not. Thinking of food in this fashion absolves me of the need for special equipment. I do not carry around a chart or calculator to figure out how much food to eat. I do not have a little book that tells me the "glycemic index" of the food I consume and I never count calories. A diet made up of a consistent variety of "real" food has the right amount of what you need on a daily basis and generalizations are quite sufficient. **Eating does not have to be academic to be healthy!**

This point was well illustrated to me when I was leafing through a nutrition book published about fifteen years ago. This particular book had analyzed food by chemical components. An apple was rated as having moderate nutritional value with only average levels of vitamins and minerals which were all listed. There was no mention of quercetin, a chemical abundant in apples that reduces allergic reactions, or all of the beneficial cholesterol-lowering fiber that comes in an apple. Similarly, berries were not given high marks because of sugar content and moderate levels of vitamins. There was no mention of the potent anti-oxidants and immune-enhancing chemicals found in berries. They were not overlooked but were just not well recognized at the time.

On a similar note, it seems that every year some new chemical is "discovered" from a natural food source and immediately hits store shelves as a supplement. Natural foods contain many different chemicals that are beneficial for our health. You do not have to wait until they are "discovered" to take advantage of these benefits. They are there all the time. We truly do live in the Garden of Eden, and you really do not have to look very hard to find it. Just pick from the wide variety of natural foods that are more abundantly available than ever before.

FOODS FROM PLANT SOURCES

An open-air market is one of my favorite places on earth. Fruits and vegetables of all colors, shapes, and sizes, all presented at their peak of freshness, just waiting for someone to place them in a bag and carry them home for supper. Which ones should you choose? *Any* and *all* of them, of course! The reds, the blues, the oranges, the yellows, the purples, and especially the greens. The colors largely come from groups of chemicals that all offer beneficial health properties. These substances are very potent anti-oxidants and are your best protection against oxidative stress, the chief factor in aging. You have probably heard of beta-carotene, lycopene, or lutein. They belong to the carotenoid family. There are over 600 different types of carotenoids, all of which have health benefits.

Beyond carotenoids, the fiber, vitamins, minerals, and other beneficial chemicals found in vegetables are important for preventing all types of disease, including cancer. Dietary fiber from vegetables, fruit, and whole grains not only improves gastrointestinal function, but also plays a large role in the removal of toxins and cholesterol from the body. Fruit pectin reduces fat absorption and removes heavy metals from the body. Enzymes present in natural foods have potent anti-inflammatory properties. The special types of fiber found in onions, leeks, artichokes and asparagus encourage the growth of favorable types of bacteria in the intestines and colon.

Admittedly, a plain stick of broccoli does not appear very interesting until you take a look at the health potential within. If everyone in the country were to eat a vegetable from the broccoli family at least once every day, the incidence of breast, prostate, and other cancers would drop dramatically! Now, that's something to get excited about. Cruciferous vegetables—which include not only broccoli but also cabbage, Brussels sprouts, kale, bok choy, and cauliflower—assist and improve the detoxification and removal of carcinogens by the liver. In addition, they increase the metabolism of hormones such as estrogen and hormonally-active toxins, thus serving an important role in preventing hormone-linked cancers.

The list of benefits from consuming vegetables goes on and on, but fortunately, you do not need to have a Ph.D. in biochemistry to take full advantage of their benefits. Mother Nature has done all of the research for you, so all you have to do is eat that bounty regularly, with as much variety as possible. For a truly healthy diet, I consider a regular assortment of vegetables to be more important than anything else.

Which types of plants we consume is now largely dictated by agriculture. More than eight thousand years of food cultivation has selected for better- tasting cultivars that provide more sugar, fat, protein and other nutrients. The overall nutritional value of many crops has been increased. Several years ago, a display at our state fair documented the evolution of the sweet potato. The "heirloom" variety (from the late 1800's) was a small, unappealing root with white meat, very different from the huge, orange, anti-oxidant-filled potatoes in markets today. Many, if not most, cultivated fruits and vegetables have followed the same course of evolution.

Over-cultivation can go too far, though, with the selection of sugar at the expense of other important nutrients and fiber. Many of our food crops have been cultivated to grow well in the non-living soil that suits the constraints of modern agriculture. Hybridization does allow us to select those qualities we find desirable in plants, but excessive hybridization has the potential to create unnatural foods that may be harmful and genetic manipulation could carry these concerns to a whole new level.

As a general rule, staying closer to what Mother Nature provides is the best way to make healthy food choices.

STEMS AND LEAVES

Of the edible plants, the parts that can be consumed vary from species to species. Roots, stems, leaves, flowers, fruits and seeds cover different aspects of nutrition, and a healthy diet includes a mixture of many diverse plants. Though they are often the least popular parts of the plant because of the absence of sugar and fat, the stems and leaves were very much a part of ancestral diets and should be held in higher regard than any other dietary component. Low in energy and protein, but very high in fiber, nutrients, and especially minerals, these vegetable parts should make up the bulk of our diet. Examples include broccoli, cabbage, celery, rhubarb, kale, spinach, collards, chard, and bok choy.

Health Tip *Many Americans have the impression that an iceberg lettuce salad is healthy food. To the contrary, iceberg lettuce offers little nutrition and is certainly in the running for one of the most flavorless foods on earth. The popularity of this type of salad has more to do with the copious amounts of meat, cheese and salad dressing placed on top than it has to do with the lettuce itself. When making a salad, opt for deep green or red lettuce. Buy organic greens if your budget possibly allows (or grow your own!). Don't hold back on the quantity, since these low-calorie vegetables are dense in nutrients.*

VEGETABLE FRUITS AND "REAL" FRUITS

When it comes to the most nutritious parts of plants, most people place fruit at the top of the food list, but because of sugar content it should really take second billing.

Less sweet fruits such as tomatoes, squash, peppers, eggplants, cucumbers and pumpkins often get labeled as vegetables, but technically anything that comes from a flower is, botanically, a fruit. For purposes of differentiation we can refer to these as "vegetable fruits" and to the better-recognized forms of fruit as simply "fruit." Vegetable fruits tend to be low in fat energy, moderately low in carbohydrates, low in protein, but high in fiber, and very high in other important nutrients; these should be our daily staples.

The sweetness of fructose (fruit sugar) is what makes real fruits so desirable but is also the factor that necessitates moderating consumption. "Temperate" fruits are seasonal fruits grown in a climate with cold winters. They are moderate in sugar, low in fat, low in protein, high in fiber and very high in nutrients. Many members of this group contain potent anti-oxidants and immune enhancers. Examples include grapes, blueberries, strawberries, raspberries, apples, pears, peaches and cherries. Different types of melons also fit in this category.

"Tropical" fruits are grown year round in warmer climates. They are higher in natural sugars than temperate fruits but low in fat, low in protein, and high in fiber and other nutrients. Examples include oranges, grapefruit, pineapples, star fruit, mangos, papaya and bananas.

Health Tip: Fruits, especially tropical fruits, are high in sugar. Yes, it is natural sugar, but it is still sugar! Concentrated fructose found in fruit drinks is more of a problem than whole fruits, but excessive consumption of fruit should be avoided. Individuals who are trying to lose weight should especially limit quantities of tropical fruits and fruit juices.

Variety is important with all foods. Too much of any one food is not a wise practice. A prime example is grapefruit. Grapefruit provides fiber and important nutrients including vitamin C, quercetin, and fruit pectin. But grapefruit also inhibits primary detoxification pathways in the liver, slowing metabolism of certain drugs, toxins and very importantly, estrogen. A recent study suggested that consuming one quart of grapefruit daily could increase postmenopausal breast cancer risk by 25-30%! (www.naturaldatabase.com)

ROOTS AND TUBERS

Many plants store energy underground. This can be in the form of an actual root or as a modified stem called a tuber. Carrots, sweet potatoes, beets and parsnips are examples of roots. Other types of potatoes such as red potatoes and baking potatoes are examples of tubers. Tubers tend to be much higher in starch. Smaller potatoes such as the red skin variety have less starch. All are good sources of minerals and nutrients, and the colors are representative of potent anti-oxidants so important for our health. As long as they do not come fried or in a box or bag, root vegetables and tubers are an important part of a healthy diet.

Almost in a class by themselves, onions and garlic should be mainstays in the diet. The chemicals that cause the pungent odors of these vegetables have anti-inflammatory, anti-oxidant, and cholesterol-lowering characteristics. Regular consumption may provide protection against heart disease, diabetes, cancer, osteoporosis and possibly even the common cold. In addition, fiber found in these root vegetables promotes the growth of favorable bacteria in the intestinal tract.

Health Tip All plants contain trace amounts of natural toxins, but the chief concern regards toxins added by agriculture. Most toxins are fat-soluble and are not retained well by the stems and leaves; therefore, they are less of a problem in "true" vegetables. The highest concern for pesticide retention is in thin-skinned fruits and vegetables that hold a lot of water. Buying organic, especially when it comes to fruits such as lettuces, tomatoes, apples, and berries, and getting to know the habits of your local farmers are wise food practices.

Down the road, we have a vegetable and fruit stand set up by a local farmer. As often as I can, I buy fresh produce there. Usually the owner is around, but sometimes I pick out what I want, weigh it myself, and place money into a slot on the top of a little metal box. Some of the produce is grown on-site, but this fellow also drives up to the state farmer's market each week to obtain more variety. He can always tell me where each item came from and when it was picked. Now and then I have the opportunity to engage him in discussions about pesticide use, living soil, global warming and the like. We do not always agree on every topic, but somehow this dirt-floored, open-air fruit stand feels more comfortable than the cold and seemingly sterile aisles of the grocery store.

SEEDS

The category of seeds includes grains, beans and nuts. A single seed is the origin of new life and thus is truly a powerhouse of nutrition. Seeds are almost (but not quite) complete packages of nutrition, containing fiber, protein, fat, carbohydrates, and other nutrients. Unlike vegetables and fruits, seeds are good sources of fat, and even more importantly, are good sources of amino acids, the building blocks of proteins. Because they are such complete foods and can be easily cultivated and stored, grains and beans now make up the majority of food for the world.

GRAINS

Grains are the seeds of grasses. The most commonly grown grains in the world are corn, rice, wheat and, distantly behind, oats. More corn is grown than any other grain, but most of it is used to feed livestock. Rice is the most widely consumed grain worldwide, but wheat is, by far, the most commonly consumed grain in the United States. All three grains have health value, but this value rapidly declines with over-consumption and excessive refinement.

Nutrition - The greatest value of grains is their resistance to spoilage. Unlike most foods that spoil rapidly, grains maintain full nutritional value for extended periods of time. The nutritional value of whole grains includes B-vitamins, protein, fiber, healthy fats and, of course, starch.

Health Tip - From a health point of view, unrefined whole grains are everything that their overly-refined cousins are not, but health attributes of whole grain products vary widely. How finely the grain is ground, type(s) of grain(s) used and the addition of other ingredients such as sugar (organic sugar is still sugar) heavily influence the health value of the final product. True whole grain products containing the complete whole grain or coarsely ground whole grain with no added ingredients are a rare find on any supermarket shelves.

Possibly one of the best examples of a true whole grain product is oatmeal, either rolled whole grain or steel-cut. Whole grain oats slow absorption of glucose, improve gastrointestinal mobility, reduce cholesterol and aid in removal of toxins from the body.

Wheat

The reason most bread is made of wheat instead of other grains is because of a special protein called gluten that allows it to rise when mixed with yeast. Wheat contains higher concentrations of gluten than any other grain and the type of gluten proteins present are the best for baking. Modern wheat (*Triticum aestivum)* has been extensively hybridized not only to increase yield but also to change gluten proteins in favor of better baking properties.

The wheat used in most pasta products is actually a different species of wheat than that used in baked goods. Often referred to as winter wheat or hard wheat, *Triticum durum* has slightly different gluten proteins and releases glucose more slowly than other forms of wheat.

Yet a different species of wheat, *Triticum compactum* is used to make pastries and cakes. This finely-ground flour releases glucose the most rapidly of all!

Health Tip Modern wheat flour is very different from the stuff your great-grandmother used for biscuits. Wheat flour typically found in modern bread and cereal products contains more starch than wheat flour from a hundred years ago—and releases glucose more readily than *nearly any carbohydrate food source, including table sugar. Oddly, whole grain flour seems to be worse than the white stuff. Wheat products alone contribute more to the epidemic of insulin resistance and diabetes than <u>any</u> <u>other</u> <u>food</u> <u>source</u>.*

Avoiding diabetes alone should enough of an incentive to reduce or even eliminate dietary wheat, but modern wheat contributes to chronic disease in other ways that go beyond glucose content alone. Intense hybridization over the past seventy-five years has actually altered the structure of the gluten proteins and transformed modern wheat into something quite different from ancient wheat. These new proteins are foreign to the human body and wreak havoc on immune function, damage the intestines and are highly inflammatory. The fiber found in modern wheat is fodder for unfriendly bacteria in the intestines, contributing to the present epidemic of bowel disease.

And anyone feeling that wheat has addictive qualities is right on target. Wheat actually contains chemical compounds similar to morphine that are mildly euphoric. These compounds stimulate appetite, induce cravings and contribute to the addictive behavior that often accompanies consumption of bread, bagels, cake, cookies and the like.

The facts that half the food products in an average grocery store contain wheat and that most Americans consume wheat products several times daily are quite concerning. After years of consuming wheat products, many people develop wheat sensitivities, typically manifesting as symptoms ranging from fatigue and arthritis to irritable bowel syndrome. Any person with any type of health concern, even just not feeling well, should strongly consider following a wheat-free diet.

There are other gluten grains, including barley, rye, kamut and spelt, but modern wheat has the highest concentration of gluten and the gluten is structurally different than gluten found in other grains. Some wheat-sensitive individuals can tolerate other gluten-containing grains.

Testing for wheat sensitivity is really not necessary: simply avoid all forms of wheat and other gluten-grains for several weeks. Improvements in well-being, intestinal function, etc., are indications of gluten intolerance. Again, gluten intolerance can be type-specific, and often other gluten grains can be added back without precipitation of symptoms. For gluten-intolerant individuals, there are many gluten alternatives and many recipe books allowing normal life without wheat or other gluten grains. Please note, however, that this is not an invitation to load up on gluten-free carbohydrates!

Wheat intolerance and wheat sensitivity should be separated from true gluten allergies. Gluten allergy, also called celiac disease, can cause a host of symptoms ranging from gastrointestinal to neurological. Gluten allergy can cause vitamin deficiencies, can mimic other medical conditions and can aggravate established medical conditions. Gastrointestinal conditions, allergy symptoms, sinusitis, arthritis, and other chronic medical conditions will often respond favorably to a gluten-free diet. Testing for celiac disease is available, but resolution of symptoms by simply avoiding gluten is generally indication enough!

Gluten allergy is forever, whereas wheat sensitivities or intolerance will resolve over time. Gluten-intolerant individuals can resume eating limited amounts of gluten after several months to a couple of years of avoiding gluten.

Rice

A daily staple for all of Asia and popular worldwide, rice is more consumed by humans than any other grain. With the wide range of varieties, rice is an exceptionally versatile food source. Fortunately, rice has not been subjected to excessive and unnatural hybridization and it is well tolerated by most people. Carbohydrate content, which partially defines the health potential of rice, is a factor of its "stickiness." White sushi rice is by far the stickiest of all rice and contains the highest concentration of starch with the lowest concentration of protein and fiber. At the other end of the spectrum, brown basmati rice is the least sticky and has the lowest concentration of starch with the highest protein and fiber. Everyday white rice leans toward the sticky end and regular brown rice leans in the opposite direction. Of course, foods consumed along with rice also affect how quickly glucose from the starch will be absorbed.

In my house, brown basmati is a staple. It has a wonderfully "nutty" flavor that blends well with many foods. Jasmine rice, another favorite, offers pleasantly fluffy texture and fragrant aroma. It is a perfect companion to Southern Asian and Indian cuisine.

Wild rice, native to North America, is actually related to cattails and not to ordinary rice, which originated in Asia. Wild rice is very high in fiber, protein and nutrients, and has a flavor all its own. For variety, it is definitely a candidate for addition to a healthy diet.

Corn

Corn claims the distinction of being the most widely produced grain in the world. Most of it, however, is not directly consumed by humans. The livestock industry commandeers the majority of corn production and the processed food industry accounts for the most of the rest, since high fructose corn syrup and hydrogenated corn oil are some of the most-used products in the commercial food industry. Whole grain corn is a good source of vitamins (especially B vitamins) and minerals. Sweet corn on the cob, whole kernels of corn in a stew, whole grain organic corn chips, and popcorn can all be included within the confines of a healthy diet.

The "big three" need to share space with all the other important grains. Grains such as barley, oats, buckwheat, rye, millet, quinoa and amaranth are becoming more available and should frequently be incorporated into a healthy diet. Each of them has its own individual health characteristics. Look for these very healthful grains in whole form or in whole grain products. They can also be bought in bulk and used in cooking for variety and taste.

Oats

Oats are definitely worth listing as a staple. They are nutritious and are well tolerated by most individuals. The unique fiber found in oats binds cholesterol and toxins for removal from the body. Though oats contain carbohydrates like any other grain, oat fiber slows absorption of glucose and prevents "sugar surges" that raise blood glucose and promote diabetes. Oats are a source of "beta-glucans," important substances known to normalize immune function. Though oats are listed as a gluten-grain, this is primarily because they are packaged and processed in facilities which mill other grains. Gluten-free oats are available (www.bobsredmill.com).

There is nothing better on a cold winter morning than steel-cut oatmeal with a little honey, raisins, and a pat of butter.

Barley

Most Americans know barley mainly for its connection with beer, where barley provides the sugar maltose, or "malt," for fermentation. Aside from use in brewing beer and feeding livestock, only a small amount of it makes it to the dinner table.

This is unfortunate, as barley is truly a wonder grain in many ways. Barley provides the highest concentration of fiber of any of the grains (13 grams per cup). The fiber in barley lowers cholesterol, raises HDL levels, and drastically slows absorption of glucose in the intestine. This is especially good news for diabetics, as blood glucose levels can actually be lowered with regular consumption of barley.

For consumption, the inedible outer hull of the barley grain must be removed. "De-hulled" barley is considered a whole grain, since the germ and bran are still present. "Pearled" barley is further processed to remove the bran, thus lowering some of the nutritional value. Barley can be eaten as a hot breakfast cereal similar to oatmeal, used as a side dish or incorporated into soups, stews and a wide variety of other dishes.

See *www.barleyfoods.org* for recipes and more information about barley as an edible grain.

Millet

Millet, known by most people as the primary ingredient of bird food, is actually an excellent grain for human consumption. In fact, millet is an ancient grain that has been consumed by humans since prehistoric times. Today, because millet is very drought resistant, it is a primary staple in dry areas of Africa. Millet is a very tasty grain and one that should be considered for dietary variety. Unlike some other grains, millet promotes growth of favorable non-fermenting bacteria in the gastrointestinal tract.

PSEUDO-GRAINS

Pseudo-grains are seeds that have grain-like characteristics, but come from broadleaf plants instead of grasses. Quinoa and amaranth, from South America, along with buckwheat, which originated in China, are now grown worldwide. These nutritious food sources offer B-vitamins, minerals, protein and fiber.

Quinoa *(pronounced "keen-wa")*

Cultivated by natives of South American for thousands of years, quinoa is just becoming known to the rest of the world. Quinoa is a complete source of protein, containing all of the essential amino acids necessary for life. Animal food sources provide a complete complement of essential amino acids, but few vegetable food sources can make this claim. Quinoa, with a taste all its own, is one of those few. It is also high in fiber, relatively low in starch, low in fat, and high in minerals.

The taste and texture of quinoa could be compared to corn grits. It cooks quickly and stores well in the refrigerator after being cooked. Quinoa can be eaten it for breakfast as a substitute for grits. "Shrimp and grits" with quinoa instead of grits is quite tasty.

See *www.quinoa.net* for recipes and more information about quinoa.

Amaranth

Easily cultivated at higher elevations, amaranth was primary food for the Incus and Aztecs. A nutritious and taste-worthy food source, consumption of amaranth is known to lower cholesterol, reduce blood pressure and improve cardiovascular function.

Buckwheat

One of the older cultivated food sources of the world, buckwheat dates back to 6000 BC in China. It was one of the first grain-like products brought to the new world and is now regularly grown worldwide. Similar to oats and barley, buckwheat contains fiber that binds cholesterol and toxins. It also slows absorption of glucose and is the most significant dietary source of D-chiro-inositol, a natural substance with known anti-diabetic effects. Though buckwheat groats (whole grain buckwheat is consumed similarly to oatmeal) take some getting used to, buckwheat waffles and buckwheat soba noodles (used in Asian cuisine) are quite tasty.

SEED SPROUTS

Young bean sprouts and newly sprouted grasses such as wheat and barley retain all of the nutritional value of the seed without the high carbohydrate content of the un-sprouted seed. The sprouting process uses up a considerable amount of carbohydrate and partially breaks down gluten, found in gluten grains. Chemicals called "lectins" found in grains, implicated as one of the inciting factors in inflammatory diseases, are also broken down by the sprouting process. Sprouted grains are high in beneficial essential fatty acids. Baked products, such as bread, made with sprouted grains have much lower levels of carbohydrate and tend to have reduced propensity to induce sensitivities; gluten sensitive individuals, however, should avoid these products.

Many people consider juices made from sprouted grass seeds to be very healthy for regular consumption. Those not enthralled with consuming a daily ration of sprouts may choose to obtain these healthy benefits from "super-green" supplements added to a daily smoothie.

Health Tip: Though bread and similar baked grain products should not be a daily affair, flour made from sprouted grains is the best choice.

NUTS

Nuts are nature's storehouse of energy and nutrition. Though there are over 300 varieties, we are generally aware of only a handful. Most commonly we think of almonds, Brazil nuts, cashews, pecans, walnuts, hazelnuts, pine nuts, pistachios, and macadamia nuts. Peanuts are actually a type of pea (legume), but they usually get thrown into the mix. Coconuts are of course a nut but seem to stand in a class by themselves.

Though we tend to think of nuts as a group, they originate from different climates, soil types, and plant types and have origins from diverse places. This allows each nut variety to contribute its own array of nutrients, including valuable minerals. Almonds are an excellent source of calcium, pine nuts are high in copper and Brazil nuts are high in selenium. In fact, a single Brazil nut will provide an entire day's allotment of that mineral—but in this case; one-a-day may be enough— too much selenium can be toxic.

> *Nutrition*   *Nuts as a group are very low in glucose, moderately high in protein, and high in favorable unsaturated fat. The fats in nuts are favorable for decreasing inflammation and are especially "heart healthy." Coconuts are the only nuts that are high in saturated fat, but the unique type of saturated fat found in coconuts is considered healthful to consume.*

> *Health Tip*   *The polyunsaturated fats in nuts easily become oxidized when exposed to air. We call such foods "stale." If nuts have a stale smell, do not eat them: oxidized fats are very unhealthy. Many packaged snack foods and snack bars (even the ones labeled as health food) are stale before you open the wrapper. I generally buy nuts fresh from a reputable source and store them in the freezer. The canned varieties are fresh, but may be loaded with salt. If you purchase nuts from open bins, make sure that they are in a cool place and that turnover is high. Fresh nuts can be reliably obtained at some grocery stores and there are many reliable nut venders on the internet.*

BEANS

"Beans, beans, they're good for your heart...." Actually, it's all true: they *are* good for your heart. High in complex carbohydrates and fiber, frijoles help remove toxins and cholesterol from the body. Beans contain chemicals called flavonoids, potent anti-oxidants that prevent plaque formation in the vessels of the heart. These same chemicals moderate the effects of reproductive hormones in disarray, thus minimizing symptoms of menopause in women and decreasing the risk of prostate cancer in men. Beans are a good source of protein. Added to brown rice or millet, beans become a "complete" source of protein providing all of the essential amino acids that we need to survive.

The list of different kinds of beans is long and includes black beans, kidney beans, pole beans, peas (many varieties), navy beans, peanuts, garbanzo beans, aduki beans, lentils, lima beans, and mung beans, just to name a few. Beans are good sources of B vitamins and some minerals, iron, calcium, potassium, and phosphorus. As with nuts, different beans provide different varieties of nutrients.

It is true that some people get increased gas with consumption of beans, but this effect tends to be more pronounced in individuals who are not regular consumers. To minimize flatulence, try rinsing canned beans before use; if using dried beans that have been soaked overnight and then drained, pour off the cooking water after it reaches a full boil, refill with water, and then cook as usual. In general, black beans, lentils, and mung beans produce less gas. An enzyme supplement can also help ease the discomfort. The problem usually improves over time with consumption of a better diet. Until then, only invite your closest friends and relatives over for dinner.

The omnipresent soybean *is so versatile that Henry Ford once made interior car parts out of them. Almost anything can be made out of soy. Considered a health food by some, use and especially overuse of soy does have some concerning aspects. Soybeans are heavily used in the commercial processed food industry as inexpensive sources of oil and protein. They are also heavily used in the livestock industry. The polyunsaturated oils are very susceptible to oxidation caused by heat. The oil is extracted using high heat and/or chemicals, making its ubiquitous use in food products somewhat concerning. The oils found in soy are "pro-inflammatory" when consumed in processed food products and contribute to increased risks of disease. Like many foods, the health potential of soy is related to whether it is whole or processed.*

Soybeans contain chemicals called "flavonoids" that act similarly to estrogen in the body. Whether this is good or bad is a matter of opinion. Products containing soy are well known to reduce menopausal symptoms in women, but this estrogenic effect has some experts concerned that flavonoids found in soy could increase risks of breast cancer. The estrogenic effect of soy, however, is extremely weak. These chemicals actually partially block the activity of estrogens that are already circulating inside the body; hence, they appear to offer protection against estrogen-induced cancers.

Possibly the greatest testament to the benefits of soy is found with the people of Okinawa, a small island off the coast of Japan. Okinawans claim the distinction of being the oldest living people on earth. Their diet includes large amounts of flavonoid compounds from soy (possibly highest in the world) and concomitantly, they have very low rates of breast and prostate cancer (possibly the lowest in the world).

The anti-cancer potential of soy is related to the flavonoid content. Steamed green soy beans, dried soy beans and tofu contain the highest levels of these important chemicals found in food sources. Soy milk contains low to moderate amounts of flavonoids. Soy sauce is low in flavonoids and processed soy oil has none. Interestingly, flavonoids only seem to be concerning when they are highly concentrated within dietary supplements. For this reason, flavonoids should only be acquired from natural dietary sources. Women who have had breast cancer should best avoid soy altogether.

Soy does have a reputation of being a "goitrogen," a substance that blocks the formation of thyroid hormones, but very likely this is a concern only with excessive consumption of soy. The incidence of thyroid dysfunction is not reported to be higher in cultures that consume large amounts of soy. Reasonable consumption of soy products should not pose a threat.

The answer to soy is the same as to any other dietary dilemma: avoid excessive use and avoid processed forms or additives. Stick with whole foods and whole food products. Steamed soybeans, which go by their Japanese name edamame, are being discovered by the rest of the world as tasty and nutritious, with a flavor somewhere between a pea and a butterbean. Tofu and tempeh, fermented soy products, are felt to offer the greatest disease-reducing benefit of any soy products. Soy sauce is one of the world's favorite seasonings and though it has a reputation for being high in sodium, low sodium varieties are available. Whole soy products are rich in essential amino acids and stand by themselves as a source of protein. They are low in glucose and low in fat but high in other nutrients.

OTHER NOTABLE SEEDS

A partial list of other seeds with the right kind of nutrition includes flax, sesame, sunflower, pumpkin and a relative newcomer on the scene—chia seeds. These seeds contain all-important essential fatty acids that moderate inflammation in the body. As with other seeds, the oils are very susceptible to oxidation and should only be consumed when fresh.

Though much attention is given to flaxseed oil for the omega 3 fatty acids it contains, whole flax seeds contain beneficial fiber and chemical substances called *lignans*. *Lignans* present in whole flaxseeds not only reduce cholesterol but also have anti-estrogenic effects felt to have value in reducing risk of both breast and prostate cancer. To gain benefit from flaxseeds, however, the seeds must be ground, or they will go right through intake, providing only a laxative effect. Consider adding 2 tablespoons of ground flaxseed to smoothies, salad or a cup of yogurt each day.

Though not as well-known as flaxseed, chia seeds offer all the attributes of flax, but are easier to keep. Chia is a dessert plant and the intact seeds are very resistant to spoilage. Chia seeds contain all of the omega-3 fatty acids, fiber and lignans found in flax, but unlike flaxseeds, the chia seeds break down immediately when exposed to water, releasing all of the internal contents of the seed in the process. A tablespoonful of chia seeds mixed in a glass of water will plump up to the appearance of tadpole eggs within minutes...and yes, chia seeds are the same seeds that were used to grow "hair" on chia pets that you remember as a child.

> **Health Tip** *If flax seeds are your choice for essential fatty acids and lignans, store them in the refrigerator. When ready for use, grind them in a portable coffee grinder and add to food. Buying pre-ground flax seeds is easier, but store them in the refrigerator and use them promptly. Chia seeds do not have to be refrigerated, unless they are pre-ground.*

SEAWEED

Seaweed is dense in anti-oxidants, nutrients, and minerals, but it is, admittedly, an acquired taste. Quality is highly dependent on the water from which it comes. Seaweed is a good source of iodine, an element often lacking in land-based diets that is important for thyroid hormone synthesis. Try a seaweed salad the next time you happen by a sushi bar. Seaweed can also be incorporated into stir-frys along with fish or shellfish. Shellfish is another excellent source of iodine in the diet.

FUNGI

The only fungi that most humans consistently consume are mushrooms and some others that make our cheese taste sharp and turn blue. Thirty years ago, mushrooms were shriveled-up, tasteless food items that only came in a jar. Now, not only are fresh mushrooms widely available but many different varieties of them are on the produce shelves. Each of them has a little different flavor, adding a signature touch to dishes. Mushrooms can impart a "meaty" flavor to certain recipes.

Nutrition *Mushrooms as a group are low in glucose and fat energy, moderate in protein, moderate in fiber and high in nutrition. Mushrooms contain chemical compounds called beta-glucans. These substances are known to normalize immune function and may play a role in reducing risk of autoimmune disease and cancer. Different mushrooms contain different types and amounts of beta-glucans. Mitake and shitake mushrooms, the best in this regard, are now commonly available.*

Health Tip *The little white variety most people are familiar with offers the least nutrition of any of the mushrooms and is colonized by a fungus that produces a toxin called aflatoxin. The fungus and toxin are destroyed by cooking; these mushrooms (and all mushrooms) should always be cooked and not eaten raw.*

FOODS FROM ANIMAL SOURCES

Animals survive by consuming plants, other animals, or both, thus repeating the cycle of life. The nutritional value of food derived from an animal source is very dependent on the nutritional value of the food that sustained that animal. For terrestrial animals, it all goes back to *living soil*. For aquatic animals, the key factor is *clean water*.

TERRESTRIAL MEAT

The two concerns associated with meat consumption are toxin concentration and the complement of fatty acids present. Large animals such as cows and hogs tend to have the highest concentration of toxins and the most saturated fat. Poultry has a higher concentration of polyunsaturated fats and retains fewer toxins. Of course, all meat is much more favorable for consumption if the animal is allowed free range to forage on grasses and other natural foods. Going even further back to our roots, meat from hunted wild animals may be the healthiest of all.

The topic of bird flu certainly makes a case for vegetarianism. Bird flu likely originated as a virus found endemically in ducks. Recent years have seen the emergence of more lethal strains of the virus that have rapidly spread into chicken and other domestic bird populations. Some people, mainly in the Far East, have apparently contracted the virus from handling birds; to date, the virus has not adapted to spreading well within human populations. The rapid spread of these lethal viruses within bird populations has been almost exclusively limited to birds confined to overcrowded, industrial-scale production facilities. The spread of disease in any animal population raised for food is always higher when overcrowding is standard procedure.

*Free-range meat is always the best choice. Some groceries are starting to carry these meats, and free-range meats of many varieties can be ordered through the Internet. The ultimate source for finding healthy meat in your region is **www.eatwild.com**.*

> **Nutrition** *Depending on the source, meat is low to high in fat, high in quality protein, and has no sugar. Beef and pork are high in saturated fat. Poultry has a higher ratio of polyunsaturated to saturated fat and is lower in fat in general, especially with the skin removed. Though meat does not provide the wealth of nutrients available in vegetables, some important minerals such as iron and selenium are present along with the important nutrients B-12, carnitine, and conjugated linoleic acid that are difficult to obtain from other sources.*

> **Health Tip** *When it comes to meat I generally stick with the real thing. Knowing what goes into processed meat foods such as hot dogs, bologna, and souse keeps them off my menu. Oxidized fat content present in these meat products contributes to diseases such as heart disease and cancer. Even hamburger has some pretty scary things ground into it and except for an occasional summer picnic, I tend to steer clear of it...and call me a weenie if you like, but when it comes to sausage, I generally save it only for special occasions or use the soy variety.*

SEAFOOD

The nutritional value of seafood tends to reflect the quality of the water from which it was harvested. A polluted body of water will definitely affect the level of toxins in the animals that come out of it. For up-to-date information about this topic in fish and shellfish, check out *www.oceansalive.org*.

Fish Fish would be the ideal source of quality protein if it were not for the mercury problem. Fortunately, many species of fish are less susceptible to this problem than others. It is an up-the-food-chain phenomenon, and, in general, large predators that feed on other larger-sized fish tend to have significantly higher mercury concentration in their flesh than fish that feed on smaller fish and crustaceans.

Nutrition Fish are high in quality protein and of course have no sugar. They are low in fat, but high in those all-important essential fatty acids. Seafood in general is high in minerals, especially less common dietary minerals such as selenium, iodine, and zinc.

Fish to avoid: Shark, swordfish, king mackerel, tilefish, tuna, sea bass, Atlantic halibut.

Fish to choose: Wild salmon, Alaskan halibut, flounder, Spanish mackerel, bluefish, grouper, light canned tuna, mahi-mahi, catfish, trout (fresh and saltwater), anchovies and—my personal favorite—sardines. (My wife makes me eat them outdoors.)

Health Tip Though farm-raised fish may be healthier than terrestrial sources of meat, aquaculture has some issues that can affect product quality. Because of the type of meal used as feed, farm-raised salmon do not have the same complement of essential fatty acids for which wild salmon are so well known. In addition, farm-raised salmon often have 6-10 times higher concentrations of toxins than those found in the wild. Avoid farm-raised crustaceans for the same reason.

Shellfish
Crustaceans Once maligned for the cholesterol they contain, crabs, shrimp, and lobster are back on the menu as healthy food items. Crustaceans are high in protein, nutrient dense, and low in glucose. Though consumption of crustaceans such as shrimp may increase LDL levels a small amount, favorable HDL levels are increased even

more. Consumption of shellfish is only a problem for individuals who have inherited a cholesterol metabolism problem (but consumption of pork or beef would be even more of a problem in these individuals). On a positive note, shrimp and their relatives tend to have high levels of favorable essential fatty acids; also, mercury contamination is not an issue here.

Bivalves   Clams, mussels, and oysters are filter feeders. They actually make the surrounding water cleaner, but they tend to concentrate any toxins and microbes in their bodies. Mollusks should only be consumed if extracted from very clean waters.

> *Health Tip* *Interestingly, this is an area where aquaculture really shines. Because feeding is not necessary, mollusks contained in special cages can be grown in pristine waters and end up being some of the healthiest seafood you can buy. Again, make an effort to know where your seafood comes from.*

Our shellfish are only as clean and healthy as the water that surrounds them. Even if you do not live near the coast, your local supplier should be able to provide information about the origins of the seafood in the market. Support your local commercial fishermen. Seafood items found in many restaurants and grocery stores are sourced from foreign markets where water quality may be alarmingly poor. You can also let your voice be heard about the quality of the seafood that ends up on your plate simply by joining grassroots organizations and supporting politicians who work for better water quality and air quality.

DAIRY

Milk is not quite the health food that commercial milk producers would have you think. Milk and milk products are high in saturated fat and lactose. Also, the dairy industry is known to use hormones to increase production and antibiotics to maintain animals in unhealthy environments. Another reason to reduce dairy consumption is the fact that most of us, as adults, lack the enzyme necessary to break down lactose (milk sugar); we call this condition "lactose intolerance."

Symptoms of lactose intolerance are primarily gas, bloating and diarrhea.

Allergies to milk proteins can also be a problem for certain individuals. Casein, the protein used in cheese production, makes up 80% of milk protein. Casein has a chemical structure similar to that of gluten and can cause problems in sensitive individuals.

Whey is soluble milk protein that is leftover as a by-product of cheese production. Whey is generally recognized as high quality protein with low potential to induce allergies. It is commonly marketed as a powder protein supplement. Whey is an abundant source of branched-chain amino acids, important for fueling working muscles.

Calcium and the Great Milk Myth: Milk is high in calcium, but whether it promotes healthy bones is widely open for debate. For years the dairy industry has held that the calcium content alone defines milk as being good for your bones, but there is little firm evidence to back up these claims; in fact, there is evidence to the contrary. North Americans and Europeans have the highest rates of milk consumption in the world—and the highest rates of osteoporosis in the world. Inversely, China has the lowest consumption of milk and milk products of any country on Earth and yet it has the lowest rates of osteoporosis of any culture. Interestingly, in Hong Kong, where milk consumption is now at European levels among the Chinese there, the incidence of osteoporosis is equal to that of European countries.

The most plausible explanation relates to blood and tissue pH. The pH of blood and tissues must be maintained at a very specific pH of 7.4 for normal metabolic functions to occur. If it varies slightly toward acidity (lower pH) or alkalinity (higher pH), the consequences are dire. Grains, meats (especially processed and aged meats) and dairy yield acid when metabolized in the body. In diets composed predominantly of acid-yielding foods (average American diet), alkalinizing minerals must be pulled from the bones to neutralize blood pH.

A lifetime of continually leaching calcium from bones to maintain normal pH almost certainly contributes to high risk of osteoporosis!

Another view suggests that large doses of calcium associated with consuming a glass of milk raise blood calcium levels <u>too</u> rapidly. In order to prevent toxic blood levels, the calcium must be removed from the bloodstream as rapidly as possible. Bone is the only place for it to go, but the excess calcium is, in effect, "dumped" into the bone, instead of being placed in a stable, organized fashion. This unstable calcium may gradually leach out of the bone, leaving holes in the bone matrix. Proponents of the theory suggests this explains the typical "Swiss cheese" appearance of osteoporosis.

For optimal utilization, consuming dietary calcium in intermittent, small amount does make sense. Non-dairy calcium sources, such as almonds, almond milk, figs and leafy greens are preferred, but certain forms of dairy may be acceptable. Yogurt is on the top of that list, along with cheese (in small amounts), and either should ideally be combined with other mineral-rich foods. The necessary amount of calcium to meet daily requirements can easily be acquired from food by most individuals.

Of course, the best solution for avoiding osteoporosis is reducing loss of calcium from bones in the first place. Vegetables provide alkalinizing minerals that help to stabilize the calcium in bones.

Yogurt is one dairy product that appears to offer significant health attributes. Yogurt is a good source of calcium, protein, and live bacteria. The bacteria break down lactose and partially digest the milk protein, resulting in a more digestible product. These bacterial cultures also contribute to a favorable bacterial balance in the large colon and vagina. Yogurt contains a substance called conjugated linoleic acid (CLA), which may inhibit cancers and decrease serum cholesterol and triglyceride. All this, and you get some calcium, too!

If you enjoy and tolerate milk and milk products, be willing to pay a little extra for organic products, free of the hormones and antibiotics used in standard milk production. For a milk substitute, consider soymilk or almond milk. Newer brands are more palatable than ever. Cooking with soymilk works quite well.

Cheese is an acceptable addition to a healthy diet, especially if excessively processed versions are avoided. (You know what I'm talking about, the kind that pours or comes wrapped in plastic and looks like plastic.) Stay with hard cheeses such as parmesan, Romano, sharp cheddar or Swiss.

EGGS

Like seeds, eggs have everything necessary to nurture new life and therefore are packed with nutrition. Eggs are important sources of certain vitamins and minerals and are an excellent source of quality protein. Eggs have high levels of lecithin, a very important ingredient for healthy cell membranes. Although they have been maligned in recent years because they are high in cholesterol, eggs also tend to be high in favorable essential fatty acids. Increased risk of cardiovascular disease and stroke need not be of concern unless you have inherited a cholesterol metabolism problem or you tend to gorge on eggs. Never forget the story of the man who won an egg-eating contest by a wide margin on one day and promptly had a stroke on the next.

At one point I was thinking that it might be nice to have a couple of hens around to provide a ready supply of our own free-range eggs. I made the mistake of sharing this thought with friends who owned a farm. Within a week a cage arrived containing one over-protective hen and five chicks. A hutch that had been constructed for a series of pet rabbits sufficed quite nicely for a chicken coop. We quickly developed a routine of letting the chickens out in the morning to forage for food and putting them back into the hutch at night. By the end of fall it was apparent that we had three new roosters and only two new hens; still, the two new hens in addition to the mother would be enough to fill our egg needs.

All went well until the mother hen began to usher her little band into the adjacent woods regularly to forage. With each visit she returned in the evening minus one chicken. Finally the mother hen did not return at all and we were down to only two roosters and zero potential for fresh eggs.

The roosters did have some aesthetic value and ate garden pests, so initially we decided to keep them around. They seemed to have gotten the idea about the woods and stayed exclusively in our yard. Within a couple of months, however, they were crowing continuously from 4 am to 4 pm and becoming a real nuisance. At first we started rooting for the local fox and hawk populations, but when they began destroying my wife's garden we began plotting their demise in earnest. We considered the hatchet; this was, after all, an ideal opportunity to obtain valuable free-range chicken meat at no cost, but the mess that would be associated with cleaning made the whole process seem unpalatable. I guess we had become too far removed from our carnivorous origins. At last a local "4-H-er" agreed to take them off our hands and we were out of the chicken business. The thought of fresh eggs from my own hens still intrigues me and this adventure may be attempted again, but for now I'll settle for eggs from a local market.

The best bet for finding healthy eggs is buying from local farmers, preferably those who have a reputation of allowing their hens to forage for food naturally and supplement with processed food only minimally. I was somewhat taken aback the first time I opened a box of true "free-range" eggs. Having been accustomed to the commercial variety—uniformly bright white, evenly sized and shaped—anything else seemed a little odd. A box of free-range eggs will often include a wonderful assortment of shell sizes and pigmentations. Egg differences do not stop at the shell: the yolks are of varying colors, all more intensely orange than those from industrial hens.

Although the taste may not be significantly different, the nutritional value very much is. Hens that are allowed to forage for natural foods produce eggs that are generally about one-third lower in cholesterol and have a much more favorable complement of essential fatty acids. The mineral content is higher and the probability of the egg harboring unwanted toxins is much lower. All in all, they are better for us and better for the chickens that produced them. A "second best" option is buying commercial eggs that are from chickens fed with organic feed that is high in omega-3 fatty acids. These eggs can be found in almost all grocery stores.

Do not make the mistake of buying eggs that are simply labeled "cage free." This only implies that the chickens are allowed to stay outside of cages. Generally it means that they live on a concrete floor and eat the same foods fed to other commercially-raised poultry. Eggs from chickens raised on organic feed are a step better, but they may not be true free-range eggs.

If it's not scratching in the yard for worms,
it's not a true free-range chicken!

MISCELLANEOUS FOOD SOURCES

OILS AND FATS

Vegetable oils are liquid at room temperature and are predominantly composed of unsaturated fats. Saturated fat and hydrogenated oils that we know of as butter, lard, and margarine are solid at room temperature.

The health potential of all types of fat depends on several variables. The enemies of oils and fat are oxygen, bacteria, heat, and chemicals used in processing. Saturated fats easily become rancid from bacterial growth, even if pasteurized. Saturated fat from animals raised under unhealthy conditions may contain toxins, hormones, and other contaminants. Vegetable oils processed with heat and chemicals are very unhealthy, especially if hydrogenated. To the contrary, both saturated and unsaturated fats from fresh, unprocessed, organic sources can be extremely healthy for regular consumption.

For the healthiest diet, a combination of different sources of fat is important, with the ideal ratio favoring unsaturated fats over saturated fats. The best sources of polyunsaturated fats are found within fresh vegetables, beans, nuts, and grains. Saturated fats are best consumed in smaller amounts such as in lean free-range meats and occasional butter used in cooking.

For cooking and oils added to food, monounsaturated oils are preferred because of their resistance to oxidation. Monounsaturated oils are excellent for cooking, dipping bread, and adding to dishes for flavor. The first on the list is *olive oil* with a wonderful flavor and the highest concentration of mono-unsaturated fat. *Macadamia nut oil* is also very high in monounsaturated fat and, of course, has a characteristic nutty flavor. *Sesame oil,* another oil high in monounsaturated fat, is stable enough for cooking and has its own unique flavor. *Peanut oil* is stable enough to be used for cooking, but has a higher concentration of saturated fat. Oleic versions (high in monounsaturated fat) of *sunflower, safflower,* and *canola oils* are excellent for cooking. Use only low heat, not high heat, when cooking with any of these oils. *Walnut oil,* higher in polyunsaturated fat, is best reserved for salads and should not be used for cooking. *Flaxseed oil* is very prone to oxidation; it should never be used in cooking and should always be stored in the refrigerator.

Picking a good oil is like picking a good wine. The label tells all. Most commercially-processed oils are exposed to high heat or damaging chemicals during the extraction process. Oxidized fat and fat damaged by heat are very unhealthy for the human body. Better quality oils will have the terms "expeller pressed" or "cold pressed" on the label. This implies that the oils have been extracted using only pressure and low heat. The very best oils will have the terms "unrefined" and "unfiltered" implying that they are even less processed and retain all of their natural nutrition. You will pay more, but the cost is worth it.

A unique oil that seems to be gaining favor these days is *coconut oil*. Once condemned because of a 90% concentration of saturated fat, coconut oil is now being raised to the level of a health food in some circles. The saturated fat in coconut is composed of "medium chain triglycerides" (MCTs for short). These fatty acids are much shorter chains than the long ones found in animal fats. Experts are suggesting that MCTs are absorbed more rapidly than other saturated fats and are much more apt to be burned immediately for energy than stored. In theory, a person could actually raise his or her metabolic energy level (and therefore lose weight) by regularly consuming MCTs. I am still of the school of thought that too much of any one thing is not a good thing, but using coconut milk in cooking occasionally is a nice way to add flavor and variety.

Another high-fat food that has gained status in recent years is the avocado. Avocados contain high levels of monounsaturated fats and are excellent by themselves or made into guacamole. A satisfactory substitute for a BLT sandwich is an ALT—avocado, lettuce, and tomato. The taste is surprisingly similar.

Life is full of compromises, and cooking with oil is one of mine. My favorite form of cooking is stir-frying, though I recognize that some damage occurs to the oil during the cooking process. I try to minimize this effect as much as possible by using only a small amount of oil and taking steps to prevent the oil from burning by only using low heat. Usually I use olive oil, but macadamia nut oil, with a natural buttery flavor, has also become a favorite. When compared to deep-fat frying, the level of health concern with stir-frying or sautéing is miniscule.

FERMENTED FOODS

More by necessity than choice, fermented foods have always been part of human diets. Edible fermented foods contribute to the normal complement of bacteria in the human GI tract, helping to insure normal gastrointestinal function. Americans consume a lower proportion of fermented foods than any culture on Earth and have higher rates of gastrointestinal problems than any culture. In Japan, about a third of the foods that make up an average diet are fermented, and, correspondingly, the incidence of lower intestinal disturbances is relatively low in the Japanese population.

Cultured yogurt is about the only fermented food that most Americans will consider eating. Yogurt is considered a "functional food" in that regular consumption of certain cultured yogurt products can be used as an adjunct for prevention and treatment of gastrointestinal disorders. Less commonly known, but also beneficial for GI function, is a cultured dairy product called kefir.

In Asia fermented foods are much more common. Examples include tempeh, a fermented soybean product common in Japan, and kimchi, a fermented cabbage product relished in Korea. Another fermented cabbage product that is a little more familiar to our European-based palate is sauerkraut. Wine, beer, and vinegar are, of course, fermented products, but they do not retain live bacteria.

Health Tip Especially for individuals who have any type of gastrointestinal disturbance, foods fermented with favorable bacteria should be a frequent dietary addition. For those who find the taste of fermented food products to be unpleasant, a daily probiotic supplement should be considered. This dietary supplement can provide the daily equivalent of bacteria found in common fermented foods.

It should be noted that not all fermentation is healthful. Many processed foods and certain uncooked foods are colonized with unfavorable bacterial and fungal species that produce harmful toxins associated with increased risk of cancer and immune suppression.

Examples of fermented foods to avoid include:

- *Sausage, bacon, salami, ham and all processed meats are often colonized with harmful types of fungi and bacteria. If they are consumed at all, they should be very well cooked.*

- *Uncooked mushrooms are colonized with fungal species and should be thoroughly washed and cooked before consumption. One of the most common toxins often associated with raw white mushrooms is called aflatoxin. Avoid raw mushrooms from a salad bar.*

- *Raw peanuts and cashews can also be colonized by fungal species, including those that produce aflatoxin.*

- *Meat from terrestrial animal sources of any kind may be colonized with undesirable strains of fungal species and should only be consumed when fresh and thoroughly cooked.*

- *Milk products including milk, cheese, ice cream, butter and cottage cheese are colonized with fungal species. Cottage cheese is by far the worst offender and should probably be avoided. Yogurt and kefir, cultured with favorable bacteria, are not colonized with fungal species.*

- *Raw eggs are colonized with fungi (and bacteria), but these are destroyed by cooking. Raw eggs should never be consumed.*

There is good and bad in everything. You can't avoid all the bad, but you can minimize your risk by being judicious about your consumption of food. Eating a wide variety of fresh foods is a wise choice.

SPICES

Spices and herbs are an excellent way to add flavor without adding extra sugar and fat. The art of cooking is truly defined by the combination of herbs and spices. They can turn an everyday dish into something special. Beyond flavor, most herbs and spices have medicinal value. Turmeric, found in most curries, is one of the most potent natural anti-inflammatory substances known and regular consumption is likely to lower your risk of cancer. Cinnamon can help you control your blood sugar, and ginger can settle your stomach when you are sick. Capsaicin, found in cayenne pepper, is another potent anti-inflammatory that is an effective topical treatment for arthritis. Garlic is an anti-microbial, anti-hypertensive, anti-coagulation, anti-cholesterol wonder food that also keeps vampires away. We could go on, but you do not have to know everything about spices to enjoy their flavor and health benefits; just toss them in.

SALT

Though Americans do tend to overuse the saltshaker, use of salt in food in this country has actually decreased over the past hundred years. Historically, salt was a primary means of preserving food. From pickles to country ham, salted food was part of every meal. As refrigeration and availability of fresh food has increased, the need to salt food has decreased dramatically. Interestingly, the incidence of stomach cancer, which was at one time a common cancer, has also declined dramatically. In Japan, where the use of salted foods is still common, the incidence of stomach cancer is significantly higher than in other developed countries.

When it comes to everyday use for seasoning food, the story on salt again appears to be another one of refined versus unrefined. Sodium and chloride ions found in shaker salt are vital for all functions within the body; sea salt includes these as well as the wide variety of trace minerals found in seawater, most of which are necessary to human health in modest amounts.

The health issue behind salt has to more with the ratio of sodium to potassium than the amount of sodium by itself. The average American diet is very low in potassium, with abundant sodium from our salty diets only compounding the problem. A diet high in vegetables is very high in potassium, with a favorable average ratio of about 5 parts potassium to 1 part sodium.

When using a salt shaker, moderate use of unrefined sea salt appears to be the healthiest option. The minerals in sea salt help maintain an alkaline pH in the blood and tissues. "Lite salt" with half sodium and half potassium is another option for those transitioning to a healthier diet.

CONDIMENTS AND SAUCES
- Mayonnaise generally contains soybean oil, eggs, vinegar, some type of sweetener, and preservatives; it is okay if only used in moderation.

Better quality spreads contain unrefined monounsaturated oils, have sugar instead of corn syrup, and use natural preservatives. Mayonnaise made with better oils such as olive oil or grape seed oil is now available.

- Salad dressings with good oils and no high fructose corn syrup are fine. Look for salad dressings with unrefined oil instead of processed soybean oil. Avoid the low-fat varieties, which tend to substitute cheap carbohydrates for oil. The best salad dressings are those that you make yourself.

- Soy sauce adds flavor to many types of dishes and is the base for many types of sauces. Look for low salt varieties or better quality brands with sea salt.

- Bottled sauces are an easy way to enhance cooking, as long as they are not used in excess. Scrutinize labels for high amounts of sugar, refined oils and undesirable preservatives. Remember, you can always make your own and put in exactly what you want.

- Ketchup, my son's favorite vegetable, has been found to contain a potent antioxidant called *lycopene*. The biggest problem with catsup is sugar, but if you are avoiding sugar otherwise, the amount in catsup does not add up too much.

- Mustard is fine as long as you can give up the hotdogs.

- Don't forget hummus—it makes a superb condiment.

- Vinegar is an excellent way to add flavor to food. Experiment with vinegars from different sources, which have interesting flavor variations.

  It turns out that vinegar is quite a health food. Consumption of vinegar daily or with meals is associated with increased absorption of calcium and strong bones, improved metabolism of glucose (decreased diabetes) and improved digestion. In fact, two tablespoons of apple cider vinegar with meals is often a cure for gastro-esophageal reflux.

BEVERAGES

Soft drinks are a natural complement to all the unnatural foods well known to a generation raised on processed food. Beyond being saturated with high fructose corn syrup or artificial sweeteners and often loaded with caffeine, these products shift the blood pH toward acidity and have a concerning link to early bone loss. There are better options for quenching your thirst.

Now an all-day beverage instead of just a morning pick-me-up, coffee has become wildly popular the Americas and Europe. Though it has a reputation for being a gastric irritant and contains significant levels of caffeine, coffee does have some chemicals that are beneficial for human consumption. The problem with coffee drinks is not the coffee itself, but the large amounts of sugar and milk fat that usually accompany them.

Most of the rest of the world drinks tea. The Asian world drinks "green tea" because the plants grow there. When Europeans discovered the beverage, they fermented the tea and dried the leaves in the sun for the long trip home. This became the "black tea" beverage to which our taste buds are more accustomed. Both forms contain anti-oxidants and other beneficial chemicals, but green tea retains a higher concentration of the original chemicals that have not been altered by the drying process. Milder and lower in caffeine than green tea, "white tea" comes from tender newly picked leaves from the tea plant. Green tea, white tea and to a lesser extent, black tea contain some of the most potent anticancer chemicals known to man and should be a regular inclusion in a healthy diet.

Tea can be made from other ingredients than the leaves of the tea plant. Herbal teas are becoming very popular and many have medicinal attributes. Chamomile and passion flower are known for relaxing qualities and ginger tea soothes the stomach. Holy basil tea has potent anti-inflammatory properties.

Many health enthusiasts turn to fruit drinks, but most fruit drinks are extremely high in fructose and should be limited. A satisfyingly fruity alternative is water with a squeeze of lime, orange or lemon and sweetened with stevia. After a vigorous session of exercise, ice-cold coconut water is very refreshing. Coconut water is a clean source of hydration that is high in potassium and provides just the right amount of sugar.

Do not forget that the basic ingredient of any beverage is plain H_2O. When you are really parched, water in its purified form quenches thirst better than anything on the planet. Of all beverage possibilities, pure water is nature's original beverage and should be consumed in greater amounts than anything else.

ALCOHOLIC BEVERAGES

Anything containing sugar can be fermented into an alcoholic beverage. The metabolites of alcohol (ethanol) are definitely classified as toxins, but alcohol does seem to have some value in small doses as an anti-anxiety agent. Red wine (and, to a lesser extent, white wine) contains potent anti-oxidants and anti-inflammatory chemicals found in skins and seeds of the grapes. Beer contains beneficial anti-oxidants as well as the vitamins folate and B6. Beer and wine both increase favorable HDL levels and decrease unfavorable LDL cholesterol levels. Numerous studies have shown that one to two 6 to 8 oz. glasses of wine daily or the same number of 12 oz. beers daily is associated with a decreased risk of cardiovascular disease, but *anything more* is unhealthy.

For some people, _any_ alcohol is too much. Know your limits. Liquor has little or no medicinal value because of higher alcohol content and because it is often mixed with other beverages containing large amounts of sugar. Even individuals who enjoy moderate use of alcoholic beverages should follow an "alcohol fast" for several weeks every so often to allow toxins to clear and systems to normalize.

SWEETENERS

What about table sugar?

Refined sugar (sucrose) is a molecule of glucose bonded to a molecule of fructose. This "double" sugar is referred to as a disaccharide. Surprisingly, table sugar contributes to a slower blood sugar rise that does pure starch. This is because the enzyme necessary for breaking the bond between these two sugars is present in the intestine, but not in saliva or in the stomach. Nevertheless, sucrose should be consumed only in minimal amounts because it still contributes to the problems of insulin resistance and diabetes.

Another concern about excessive consumption of disaccharides such as sucrose and lactose (milk sugar) is their effect on intestinal bacteria. Disaccharides can cause alterations in the balance of bacteria in the colon, contributing to disorders such as irritable bowel syndrome and overgrowth of yeast in some individuals. Though more common with disaccharides, any sugars (including high fructose corn syrup) can cause overgrowth of unfavorable bacteria in the gut. Imbalances in intestinal flora (gut bacteria) can have wide-ranging, adverse effects. Autism and attention-deficit disorder both have strong ties to microbial gut imbalances.

Refined sugar, in the amounts consumed by most Americans, is a major contributor to America's health problems, but like many things, sugar is only a problem if used excessively.

Natural sweeteners such as honey, maple syrup, and agave nectar add pleasure and flavor to food. These sweeteners do contain fructose and glucose, but the potential for harm is defined by the amounts used. With conservative use, these products can be enjoyed in tea, yogurt, oatmeal or wherever just a touch of sweetness is indicated.

Honey provides glucose and fructose derived from sucrose found in the nectar of flowers. The sucrose is broken down by enzymes inside bees. Honey offers much more than sugar. A wealth of nutrients derived from flower pollen including vitamins, minerals, enzymes, anti-microbial substances, and other essential nutrients are found within honey. Honeys with the most health benefits are not cooked and come from mixed varieties of wildflowers, as opposed to the more common monoculture varieties such as clover. Some people have found that regular consumption of honey derived from local flowers prevents seasonal allergies.

Maple syrup is another natural sweetener not to be overlooked. Beyond flavor, maple syrup offers B vitamins and minerals, especially zinc.

Agave nectar is sweeter than sugar, low in glucose, but high in fructose. Its flavor is less distinct than honey or maple syrup, providing another alternative for sweetening beverages or cereal.

And artificial sweeteners?
Saccharin has been around the longest. It has an aftertaste and carries that lingering concern associated with cancer studies in laboratory animals. It is probably one best to be avoided.

Aspartame (NutraSweet) consists of two amino acids, aspartic acid and phenylalanine, joined in a way that touches our taste buds for sweet. Many diet soft drinks and a host of other products contain aspartame. Aspartame is not heat tolerant and therefore cannot be used in cooking. Individuals who cannot metabolize phenylalanine must avoid the product completely. There seem to be some concerns surfacing regarding symptoms related to chronic intake of aspartame. Excessive aspartic acid and phenylalanine could cause imbalances in serotonin and other neurotransmitters, which may contribute to depression and other neurological symptoms. Aspartame is approved by the FDA as a safe substance but excessive use should be avoided.

Sucralose (Splenda) is the newest arrival on the artificial sweetener scene. This product is 600 times sweeter than table sugar (sucrose). Sucralose is derived from cane sugar, but three of the oxygen atoms in the sucrose molecule are then replaced with chlorine atoms. This creates stronger chemical bond that is not broken down by enzymes in the human body. According to the company, sucralose is non-toxic, is eliminated unchanged in the feces, does not affect insulin levels, and can be used anywhere that regular sugar would be—even by diabetics.

While the safety statistics presented by the company look good, it's still too early in the game to tell for sure. In my opinion, any substance that isn't natural to the human body has at least some potential for harm. Strong chlorinated chemicals are used in manufacturing and I wonder how much residual chemical is left behind. I also wonder about how efficiently sucralose is completely removed from the body.

Stevia is a natural alternative that is functionally similar to sucralose. Stevia is an extract of leaves of a plant native to South America. It has been used by humans there for over a thousand years. The sweetening capability of the plant comes from several molecules of glucose fused together in a way that cannot by broken down by the human body.

Stevia has recently been approved as food additive and is showing on supermarket shelves with other sweeteners. The only "side effects" noted with Stevia are lowered blood sugar and reduced blood pressure! Stevia has been used in Japan for over thirty years. There are several cookbooks available for cooking with Stevia. Look for *Stevia Sweet Recipes* by Jeffrey Goettemoeller.

Xylitol is not yet well known, but may be one of the better options for a sugar substitute. *Xylitol* is a sugar-alcohol found naturally in berries, plums, mushrooms, and corn husks. It is as sweet as sucrose, but only carries 1/3 the calories. There is no aftertaste. Xylitol is absorbed more slowly than glucose and has less impact on insulin levels, thus it is safe for diabetics. An interesting feature of xylitol is that it appears to prevent tooth decay and reduce plaque. There is some evidence that regular consumption may have a favorable effect on bone density. At present there is no known toxicity.

My greatest concern about sweeteners such as sucralose, Stevia and even xylitol is the possibility of tissue damage from adherence to proteins or unknown effects on chemical messengers in the immune system. Theoretically, Stevia and sucralose pass through the intestines unchanged with little or no absorption, but I'm not completely convinced. Xylitol is broken down, but is not regulated by insulin and could, theoretically, contribute to "protein-sticking."

Life almost demands a bit of sweet now then, just not in the amounts used by most people on a daily basis. The best overall strategy is small amounts of a variety of sweeteners, with table sugar sometimes included. Stevia does appear to have some health benefits and I recommend it, just not excessively or exclusively.

CHOCOLATE

What can I say? For some of us, chocolate is an essential ingredient for life. I could not start my day without a lump of dark chocolate. Besides being delicious, chocolate contains anti-oxidants and other chemicals that are beneficial from a health point of view. It seems to be a natural mood elevator. There is also good evidence that a small amount of chocolate, consumed on a daily basis, is associated with lowered blood pressure in individuals with hypertension. The recommended daily dosage is 1-2 oz. of dark chocolate with at least 60% cocoa content.

For more extensive information on food and food sources, spend some time at the following websites:

www.localharvest.org
www.organicconsumer.org
www.whfoods.com

CHAPTER 8

Healthier Food, Healthier Eating

Changing to a healthier way of eating is a real challenge, especially if it means going against the established norm. Often, it's like paddling upstream against the current, while everyone else is happily floating downstream, seemingly oblivious to the rapids just around the bend. Overcoming personal cravings is one thing, but doing something different than everyone else around you is truly difficult, all while the commercial food industry is constantly trying to lull you into a comfort zone of being happy with what they provide.

In the last chapter and in this one, I have provided solid information and guidelines for individuals interested in making a real change. These guidelines are drawn not only from present day knowledge about nutrition, but also from what our past dictates a healthy diet should be. For those willing to paddle upstream, the rewards are great!

GUIDELINES FOR CHOOSING HEALTHY FOOD

1. Choose unrefined whole foods, avoiding processed foods. The health potential of food is defined by how close it is to its natural origins. Any food loses nutritional value with processing. Commercially processed foods are low in nutrition and are the chief source of excessive dietary glucose, abnormal fats, and toxins that define an average American diet. The first and most important step in changing to a healthier diet is getting rid of them.

We could stop right here and make this our one and only rule of healthy food, but life is not so straightforward. Can you imagine if you had to make everything from scratch, right down to the ketchup? Even then, some processing would be inevitable, as cooking is a form of processing. The question becomes this: how much and what types of processing are we willing to accept?

Time is the issue. If we each had an abundance of free time and a flare for creative cooking, healthy foods would grace every meal. Few of us have this luxury. The pace of life today makes the goal of cooking meals very challenging.

The solution is finding creative ways to fit whole foods into a busy American lifestyle and being very selective about which commercially available products we buy. The FDA has helped us out in this respect by requiring the commercial food industry to tell us what is in our food. Information about fiber content, carbohydrates, fat and protein, vitamins and minerals are included, along with a list of specific ingredients for all packaged foods. Most importantly, the ingredients contained within the product are listed in decreasing order by weight.

When using packaged or bottled products, get into the habit of reading labels, but remember that the majority of the daily diet should be made up of foods <u>without</u> labels.

Below are some "red flags" to look out for when scrutinizing package labels.
- **Any food items that contain any of the threatening three:** *wheat flour (white or whole grain), high fructose corn syrup,* or any *partially hydrogenated oil* should be strictly limited or avoided completely. This means that cookies, pastries, doughnuts, white bread, potato chips, and the like all have to go.

Unfortunately, it's true—maintaining an ideal weight and a healthy body is virtually impossible with consumption of these food products!

- **Any food product that contains chemical additives that you do not recognize should be avoided.**

- **In general, any food product with more than six ingredients on the label should be scrutinized carefully.**

- **My advice for counting carbohydrate and fat calories is specifically not to.** Whole foods have the correct amount of what you need, in the correct ratios. Whole foods have healthy carbohydrates and healthy fats that do not need to be counted. Put away the calculator and the notebook and start eating right!

The glycemic index, which is a measure of the tendency of a given food to release glucose, has value but should not be relied on absolutely. Most foods are rarely consumed in an isolated fashion, and combining foods dramatically affects the overall glycemic index of the meal. For example, vegetables, beans, barley, or oats slow the absorption of high glycemic foods such as carrots or red potatoes when they are eaten together.

Following a healthy, whole foods diet obviates the need for any type of calculations!

- **Avoid processed meats of *any* variety.** The hotdogs and bologna have to go. For so many reasons, they are just downright unhealthy.

AGEs, the protein-sticking complexes that directly contribute to aging and disease, can also come from sources outside the body. Processed meat and meat that has been fried at high temperatures contain AGEs. When these products are consumed, externally-acquired AGEs accumulate in the same way that they accumulate from carbohydrate consumption.

- **Avoid refined oils and products that contain refined oils.** Refined oils are liquid at room temperature and have not been hydrogenated, but the high heat and/or chemicals used in the extraction process create oxidized fats. Finding them in food is not always straightforward, since refined oils are hidden in everything from mayonnaise to salad dressings. At better quality groceries and health food stores look for "unrefined" oil on product labels.

- **Do not eliminate food groups.** Eating a wide variety of foods containing a mix of nutrients is important. Avoid strict low-carbohydrate or low-fat diets. Eating fats and carbohydrates that are healthy is important, and eating whole foods helps ensure that you get the correct balance. Avoid products labeled as "low-fat" such as salad dressings and mayonnaise; these products substitute poor-quality carbohydrates for fat and generally have more of a detrimental effect on blood lipids and blood glucose. Try using smaller amounts of the regular variety.

- **It's a matter of time.** Commercially-prepared or processed food is nothing more than a time-saving device. For processed foods to be acceptable, they should equal the same product made at home using whole food ingredients. Even so, anything made fresh from scratch is going to be healthier.

- **Be aware of the new wave of "healthy" processed foods.** New items with sensational labeling are showing up in both regular groceries and health food stores. From olive oil potato chips and natural health food bars to vegetarian lasagna and organic breakfast cereals, healthy is in style. To their credit, these products use organic flour, organic sugar, and non-hydrogenated oils, but still have the problem of excessive glucose and low nutrition. A sniff of that "healthy" granola bar will reveal a slightly stale smell that is indicative of oxidized fat. Granted, some of these foods are probably better than their alter egos, but they should not make up the lion's share of what you eat each day. They still fit into the commercially processed food category that generally should be restricted.

- **Be aware that the commercial food industry is more interested in your money than your health.** They are in the business of selling what sells. If health happens to sell, the better for everyone, but be particular about what you buy. The chief concern of any business selling food is the bottom line. Even "healthy" foods often contain fillers to bring down the total cost. For example, packaged organic vegetable lasagna contains mostly noodles, sauce, and cheese with a meager amount of vegetables. It is twice the price of typical packaged frozen lasagna and is probably not much healthier.

2. **Eat your vegetables!** The nutritional question posed really does not matter; the answer almost invariably is "eat more vegetables!" Vegetables provide antioxidants, nutrients and healthy fats. High in fiber, vegetables are essential for reducing toxins and cholesterol and also for slowing absorption of glucose. That same fiber supports

friendly bacteria in the gut. Minerals provided in vegetables buffer pH. Regular consumption of vegetables lowers risk of all diseases and slows the processes of aging. The health of your diet is directly proportional to the amount of vegetables it contains—the more variety, the better. No vitamin pill can come close!

Vegetables and fruits should account for 50% or more of your total daily diet.

Strive to eat a higher proportion of vegetables by volume than anything else. For individuals who have not learned to enjoy the flavor of vegetables, this is a tall order. Spices, seasonings, and creative dishes can help you accomplish this goal. Start with vegetables you know and like. Regularly incorporate them into meals.

As an exercise in eating healthily, each week pick a new vegetable that is unfamiliar. Do an Internet search for recipes that contain that vegetable. Look for recipes which incorporate the new vegetable with other foods, so that the flavor is not overwhelming. After a while, new flavors and new foods will become enticing instead of threatening.

3. **An apple a day...** Try to eat an apple, a peach, a plum, a slice of melon or a handful of some type of berries every day. Red grapes, blueberries, cherries, blackberries, and other types of berries contain potent ant-oxidants. Add them to yogurt, or just eat them plain. Follow the seasons when different types of temperate fruits are available, but frozen or dried will do in the colder months when nothing fresh is at hand. Variety is a key principle for all food sources.

4. **Whole grains are whole foods.** Completely avoiding grain is not only difficult but is unwarranted. Whole grains offer considerable nutritional value. They offer a healthy source of carbohydrates, vitamins and minerals, and are typically high in fiber. Grains such as oats, brown rice, and barley should be considered a standard part of a healthy diet. Once in a while, try an unfamiliar grain such as millet, teff, or quinoa—the Internet is full of recipes!

    Having said this, however, grains should be consumed in moderation; they should not replace vegetables as the primary source of food. Whole grains of any type are still high in carbohydrates and if consumed in enough quantity can contribute to insulin-resistance and obesity. Wheat (white flour and whole grain flour alike) and <u>refined</u> corn products should be limited (and some cases avoided). Bread and pasta, even though they hit all the right taste buds, should be an occasional treat instead of a daily affair. Sprouted grain products offer a healthier alternative.

Wheat and gluten intolerances are common. If health problems are present, consider following a strict gluten-free diet for a period of six weeks. Improved gastrointestinal function or reduction in symptoms such allergies and pain associated with arthritis is evidence of gluten intolerance.

Gluten-free flours, mostly containing tapioca, potato, cornstarch and rice starch, are often substituted for wheat flour, but have just as much propensity to contribute to insulin resistance and diabetes—save it for special treats. Buckwheat, whole-grain oat and teff flours do not release glucose as rapidly and offer other health benefits.

5. **Eat more beans!** Beans contain high quality protein, are generally low in fat, and provide complex carbohydrates that do not adversely affect blood glucose; in fact, beans slow the absorption of glucose from other foods. They are also high in fiber and contain antioxidants and other chemicals that may prevent cancer and atherosclerosis. Beans come in a wide variety of flavors, shapes, colors, sizes, and can be incorporated into a wide assortment of dishes or eaten alone. Hummus is excellent as a mayonnaise-substitute on sandwiches, as a thickener in dishes, and as a dip for raw vegetables.

6. **Don't be afraid to snack on nuts.** Nuts contain favorable types of fats and are a good source of protein and important minerals. They satisfy hunger without raising blood sugar. Look for raw or low salt varieties. Nut butters are a good snack food and make excellent thickeners in dishes. Try some varieties other than peanut butter. Nuts and nut products are high-calorie foods, however—a factor that should be taken into consideration if trying to lose weight! A variety of nuts can be a regular part of your diet.

7. **Humans are omnivores and meat has always been on the menu.** Fresh lean meat including seafood and terrestrial sources obtained wild or raised "grass-fed" can certainly be included as part of a healthy diet. Even with healthier meat, however, consumption should be appropriately limited. It is time for meat to step out of the spotlight for

a change. Use meat within a dish or as a side-dish, rather than as the main course. Small amounts of meat can be used to add flavor to dishes that are predominantly vegetable. Poultry and seafood are preferred over beef and pork. As a general rule of thumb, meat should make up 10% or less of your total food. Only about 3-6 oz. of lean protein per day is essential.

8. **Compromise as needed with the use of dairy products.** Lactose intolerance and milk-protein allergies are common. People with any kind of gastrointestinal problems, allergy problems, or chronic inflammatory disorders should probably avoid milk products altogether. Yogurt is an exception to the rule, as most people can tolerate cultured yogurt. Those who tolerate milk and milk products can include low-fat organic milk and cheese in moderation. Cottage cheese should be avoided due to potential aflatoxin contamination.

    Plain, low-fat yogurt is a good snack food, especially when combined with fresh berries and nuts. Plain yogurt is also excellent for adding a creamy taste to recipes in place of cream or sour cream. Other fermented foods are acceptable on a daily basis. If you do not have a taste for any fermented foods, a daily probiotic supplement is recommended, especially if gastrointestinal disturbances are present.

    Goat's milk products, if you can adjust to the flavor, are more easily digested.

9. **Strong bones.** While the verdict is still out as to whether milk consumption is wise, there are other excellent dietary sources of calcium: tofu, nuts (especially almonds), beans (soybeans, chick peas and mung beans), figs, kelp, collards, broccoli, kale, okra, chocolate(!) and fish (especially sardines, salmon and scallops).

    Maintaining a slightly alkaline pH in blood and tissues is the best way to keep calcium and other minerals in bones. The natural way to maintain alkaline pH is by adhering to a high vegetable diet, free of processed and refined foods. The minerals in sea salt may also help maintain alkaline pH.

10. **A fish a day?** Centuries ago, we would have all done well to eat some type of oily fish every day. In these times, however, with mercury contamination of large fish and water pollution being ever-present concerns, we need to carefully consider our seafood choices. Follow the

suggestions in the "food classification" section for safe consumption of fish and seafood. Eating seafood at least twice a week under these circumstances is a reasonable practice.

The evidence in favor of a daily fish oil or essential fatty acid supplement is quite strong, especially in individuals over age 40. Choose a quality supplement that is free of any contaminants or oxidation. A high quality supplement should not have a fishy taste or odor. Supplements are available that blend a variety of essential fatty acids from both vegetable and marine sources.

11. **Eggs can be a dietary staple.** Consumption of somewhere between two and six eggs per week is perfectly reasonable. Eggs from organic "free range" chickens are high in omega-3 essential fatty acids and are worth the extra money. As always, moderation and variety are the key words.

    Abnormal cholesterol is more related to excessive carbohydrate consumption than to consumption of foods containing cholesterol. Except those with a family history of hypercholesterolemia, most people can eat eggs with little concern.

12. **Salt.** When adding salt to food, choose unrefined sea salt. Life originated in the sea and the trace minerals present in sea water are important for all living things. Avoid salted meats and pickled foods. Limit salted, processed and packaged food such as chips. Use low-sodium soy sauce.

13. **Spice up your food!** Spices not only make food more interesting and add flavor without adding extra sugar and fat, they also make food healthier. Many of the spices and herbs have anti-inflammatory properties and virtually all of them have some positive medicinal value.

14. **Balance the oils and fat in your body.** Poly-unsaturated fat should come mainly from natural foods and not added oil. Oils used for cooking and added to food should be un-refined and predominantly mono-unsaturated. A small amount of saturated fat and cholesterol found in natural food is actually healthy for consumption.

15. **Getting enough protein.** Proteins make up the machinery and structural components of the body, and every day, old proteins are broken down and replaced with new. A complete protein source is one that provides

all of the essential amino acids. Meat, eggs, and dairy are complete sources. Soybeans are also complete sources of protein. Combinations of foods that do not by themselves provide all of the essential amino acids can be complete sources of protein. An example would be combining brown rice with beans.

Americans seem to be obsessed with getting enough protein. It is true that we need to consume enough protein to account for the daily turnover of amino acids in the body, but this amount is easy to acquire. We really do not need more than this amount. In fact, consuming large amounts of protein is hard on the kidneys and can be toxic. High animal protein diets push the pH of the body toward acidity which must be balanced by leaching minerals from bones (increasing risk of osteoporosis). The dietary recommendations in this chapter more than allow for an adequate amount of quality protein.

16. **Drink plenty of water.** Clean, pure water should be your primary beverage. Strive for a couple of liters every day. Green or white teas with minimal sweetening are the best options for flavored beverages.

17. **To cook or not to cook.** Some individuals advocate strict raw food diets, but light cooking helps break down food, releasing enzymes, vitamins and nutrients. Also, cooking destroys toxins produced by fungal species and unfavorable bacteria that colonize many food sources. Heated food, especially in winter, encourages the enzymatic processes of digestion and warms the body.

Raw foods in the form of salads, cut vegetables, and occasionally sushi are perfectly acceptable, but do not necessarily need to form the majority of your diet. The normal practice of consuming salads at the beginning of the meal actually makes sense. Raw foods very likely provide natural enzymes that aid in digestion of other foods.

Juicing is a healthful way to obtain all the benefits of fruits and vegetables without having to consume a large volume of fruits and vegetables. Health benefits, however, are very much dependent on what goes into the juicer. Organic and fresh are the by-words for juicing. Fruits and vegetables have the potential to contain both natural and synthetic toxins. Some fruits are very high in sugar. Fresh frozen is acceptable if not freezer-burned. Vegetables and temperate fruits such as berries should be the main source of the juice.

When it comes to cooking, steaming is by far the healthiest mode. Steam breaks down fiber, renders food more digestible and seals in nutrients. Steaming does not destroy natural enzymes found in food. Baking is fine, but takes time. Stir-frying and sautéing are tasty ways to seal in nutrients, but have the disadvantage of adding heated oil—using only low heat is the key to keeping it healthy. Grilling seals in nutrients and removes some fat, but adds toxins in the form of smoke and char. Avoid charring as much as possible when food is on the grill. Boiling is not an ideal form of cooking because nutrients are leached from food. The verdict is not yet final on microwave cooking. It would seem to be similar to steaming, but there are suggestions that microwaves may adversely change the structure of chemical nutrients within the food. Overcooking should always be avoided, with the exception of meat which should be cooked through and through.

Deep-fat frying is the only method of cooking that should be discouraged completely. It is true that deep-fat frying is the ultimate marriage of glucose and fat and that anything, even shoe leather, coated in flour and dropped into a deep fat fryer for several minutes tastes good; nevertheless, deep-fat frying is a true health hazard.

Before about 1900 acquiring enough fat to use for deep-fat frying was very expensive. The abundance of grain has brought with it a cheap source of vegetable oil, such that deep-fat frying has now become a staple in fast-food restaurants. This method of cooking may hit all the right taste buds, but fried foods are major contributors to the obesity problem, cardiovascular disease, and cancer. In my opinion, the only good thing that comes out of frying food is the leftover oil, which can be converted into biodiesel to fill the tank of your car and help conserve our precious petroleum supplies!

18. **Fresh is best.** Excessive cooking and excessive processing quickly decrease the nutritional value of food. Age and spoilage allow the growth of toxin-producing fungal and bacterial species. For most foods, fresh is best. Fresh frozen is almost as good. Avoid excessive use of foods containing preservatives. Fish, beans and tomatoes retain most of their beneficial nutrients when canned, but most vegetables do not. We live in a time when fresh food and refrigeration are readily available. Take advantage of it.

19. **Select food that has origins in living soil (organic food).** Industrial-scale production of food depletes minerals in the soil and therefore decreases the nutritional value of the harvest. Foods produced using chemical pesticides, hormones, and antibiotics also have obvious health concerns. We all pay the costs in the long run—with our health and in damage to the environment.

The Environmental Working Group (www.ewg.org) has set up simple guidelines for choosing organic vegetables and fruit.

Dirty Dozen*: peaches, nectarines, apples, pears, celery, sweet bell peppers, imported grapes, berries in general, spinach, lettuce, potatoes and tomatoes.*

Clean Fifteen*: onions, avocados, frozen sweet corn, pineapples, mangos, asparagus, frozen peas, kiwi, bananas, cabbage, broccoli, papaya, melons, sweet potatoes and eggplant.*

With other fruit and vegetables, organic is preferred if price and availability allow. Choose organic whenever buying packaged goods such as grains, nuts, soymilk, almond milk, or dairy products.

Strive for 75% organic!

20. **Support your local farmer and the local vegetable stand down the road.** Produce purchased from a familiar face is pleasant and comforting. It may not be organic, but many small farmers are using better farming practices and fewer chemicals than mega-agriculture. All you have to do is ask!

One step further is growing your own. Having a small garden is pleasing in many ways and may be the way to have the healthiest food around.

See *www.localharvest.org* for information about finding local food sources.

21. **The high cost of food?** Cost is always relative. Americans like their food quick and cheap, with little concern for quality, but the cost of cheap food goes well beyond what you pay at the grocery store. Presently America spends only about 7% of the gross national product (GNP) on food. We spend 15% of the GNP on healthcare. The math behind the real cost of better food is simple. If we were to spend twice as much on healthier food, very likely we would spend only half as much on healthcare costs, thus breaking even. And this estimation does not

even include the environmental costs of producing cheap food that we all pay for in the long run. When all variables are added in, better quality food is not only cost-effective but also offers a better life for everyone. *Loosen up your pocketbook: you deserve better food!*

The high cost of food is often more about the high cost of convenience than the actual cost of food. Even the priciest grocery stores have a good supply of raw food products (rice, beans and such) at very reasonable prices. Whole vegetables, in season, are generally not expensive. Meat is generally the most expensive item in the grocery cart, but cutting back on meat consumption is a good practice anyway. Organic, free-range meat costs twice as much as the grocery store variety, but if you eat half as much, the cost is the same. Organic whole grain oats, barley and rice are not expensive. Dried beans are cheap.

A fancy container of hummus costs as much as $4.50, but enough garbanzo bean flour (or canned garbanzo beans), tahini, and other ingredients to make about 10 containers of hummus costs about $15.00 ($1.50 each)—and it's easy to make. A batch of quality hummus only takes about 30 minutes to prepare.

Remember, the closer you get to the source, the more you control the quality and flavor of the end product.

22. **Variety is the spice of life**. There are many reasons why variety is important, but, first and foremost, it is essential for providing adequate nutrition. No single food source is complete. Consuming a wide variety of foods increases the probability of obtaining all of the vitamins, minerals, fiber and other nutrients necessary for good health.

   Even foods we consider "healthy" are not perfect. Most food has at least some potential for harm. It may be a hidden toxin or potential to cause sensitivity in some people. Negative aspects of consuming a certain food could add up over time. Rotating foods and enjoying variety reduces this likelihood.

23. **Normal pH balance.** Enzymes in the body function optimally when the blood and tissues are at a slightly alkaline pH of 7.4. The body has complex buffering systems that normally guarantee maintenance of this specific pH, and only in states of severe disease does the pH of blood and tissues waiver.

Metabolic processes in the body are continually generating acid. Certain foods, including grains, meat, and dairy, yield acid when metabolized in the body. The body must constantly neutralize acidity to maintain normal pH. Mechanisms for balancing pH include removing acid via the kidneys and lungs, as well as neutralizing acid by adding alkalinizing minerals. Vegetables and certain other foods provide alkalinizing minerals that neutralize acidity. If alkalinizing foods are not present, the body must pull calcium salts from bones to ensure a stable pH.

Continually leaching calcium from bones to neutralize acid appears to be a significant contributing factor to osteoporosis. Regularly consuming foods that push the pH toward acidity may also be a factor in the formation of stones in the kidneys, bone spurs, and calcium deposits at other locations in the body. Deposits of these minerals form when excessive acid is neutralized. Deposition of uric acid crystals in joints associated with gout is driven by this same process.

If you have spent your life leaching minerals from your bones, putting them back is not going to be easy. Medical therapy is sometimes indicated, but you can start slowing the loss right now by changing your dietary and lifestyle habits!

Common foods considered to have a positive alkaline effect include **virtually all vegetables**, pumpkin seeds, flax seeds, coconut oil, olive oil, sesame seeds, almonds, avocado, lima beans, white beans, lentils, tofu, garlic, mushrooms, Stevia, sea salt and alkalinized water. Alkaline grains include buckwheat, quinoa, millet, spelt and sprouted seeds.

Most fruits are mildly acidic, but provide alkalinizing minerals when metabolized, so are considered neutral or mildly alkaline. Bananas, though high in sugar, are alkaline.

The main foods considered to have an acidic effect include soft drinks, wheat, corn, oats, refined sugar, rice, dairy products, all meat and meat products, refined oils, artificial sweeteners (especially aspartame) and alcoholic drinks.

Some foods that offer health benefits are found in the acidic list. The recommendation does not imply that these foods should be avoided, but that total diet should be weighted toward alkalinity.

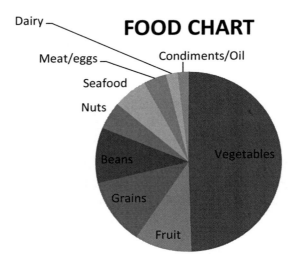

FOOD CHART

THE GREAT REFRIGERATOR AND PANTRY MAKEOVER

An exercise for learning about food starts in your own home. After thoroughly digesting the information and guidelines on food and eating, remove all food items from the refrigerator, cabinets, and pantry. (No, it doesn't have to be done all at one time and yes, it was high time for it anyway!) Create two separate areas in each of the places you store food. Items that would be classified as "acceptable" according to the food guidelines are placed in one area and everything else in the other area. In most homes the "acceptable" pile is going to be rather small at first (but hopefully not non-existent). Gradually change the ratio until the "un-acceptable" items are an insignificant part of the pantry and 'fridge. Every couple of weeks re-read the guidelines to monitor progress. You are on your way to having a healthier diet and living a healthier life!

TIPS FOR BETTER EATING HABITS

1. **CHEW YOUR FOOD THOROUGHLY AND COMPLETELY.** The digestive system works better if it has time to digest and if food is well chewed before it is presented to the stomach. Chewing food thoroughly causes you to eat slower. Eating slower allows time for the normal physiological signals that gradually reduce hunger and allow a feeling of satiety. Chewing food thoroughly is also a first step in alleviating any sort of gastrointestinal problem.

   For most of us, chewing takes practice. We live in a world where gulping down food on the run is the norm. Eating slowly and chewing thoroughly takes practice. With time, chewing more slowly should become an unconscious effort.

   Following a rapidly consumed meal with a large cold drink also is not a good idea from a digestion point of view. Liquid consumed in large amounts during or immediately after a meal dilutes enzymes necessary for proper digestion. Cold liquid slows enzymatic processes and gastric motility even further.

   This one was really tough for me. I have always eaten very rapidly and for most of my life I consumed large quantities of iced tea or soft drinks with every meal. I am just starting to be able to slow down enough to savor meals and often have hot tea or just a glass of water without ice. Sipped wine or beer is also a natural accompaniment to food.

   Make an attempt to sip a beverage that accompanies a meal, rather than gulping several drinks. If you are thirsty, drink your beverages well before beginning the meal. Room temperature liquids are more ideal than iced beverages.

2. **Portion size matters.** Statistically, long life is much more associated with eating less than anything else. Even so, living life with chronic hunger pangs is not a necessity to be healthy. Most people chronically eat more food than they actually need and continue eating until they are completely stuffed. Often we eat food not because we're hungry, but because it's there. Before putting food into your mouth, get into the habit of asking yourself: *Do I really need those calories? Am I really hungry? How much of that special treat do I really need to be satisfied?*

   Make a pledge to stop eating before you are 80% full. Eating more slowly and chewing food thoroughly is an automatic way to learn to eat less food. Filling up on vegetables instead of starches and sugar is a good practice. *Another helpful tip is using smaller plates and bowls.* The perception of a full plate goes a long way towards relieving hunger, though a smaller plate doesn't warrant refilling it repeatedly.

3. **How often should you eat?** It probably does not matter—whatever feels comfortable is the right answer. Most experts are now recommending five to six small meals a day. Contrary to that opinion, I have met plenty of folks in their nineties who owe their longevity solely to the fact that they typically eat only one meal a day. *The type of food seems to be more of an issue than the frequency of eating. High intake of vegetables is directly associated with improved longevity and better health.* Insulin-resistant individuals (most people reading this) tend to best tolerate small, frequent meals until insulin levels gradually return to normal.

   Personally, I like to start my day with breakfast. It gets me going in the morning. Throughout the day I will generally have several low calorie snacks and one other full meal. Whenever it comes during the day, a full meal should be a relaxed event.

4. **A word of caution about changing to a healthier diet.** Let's face it: by the time they get around to changing to a healthier diet, many people are not very healthy. This includes the gastrointestinal tract. Gastrointestinal dysfunction is caused by poor dietary and eating habits. Normal gastrointestinal function is essential for digestion of the complex foods found in a healthy diet. When they first change their diets, people who are not used to healthy food will often initially notice that symptoms of bloating and gastric discomfort actually increase. Do not worry—these symptoms should gradually resolve. A healthy diet encourages healing and generally, with time, gastrointestinal function improves.

   Consider supplementation with probiotics and digestive enzymes to aid in digestion of newer and more complex foods when you are making an abrupt diet change.

5. **It's only human to cheat every now and then.** Make an "exceptions list" for foods that are decidedly unhealthy but are difficult to leave behind.

My father makes the best peanut brittle in the world, a perfect crunch made from real butter, raw sugar, and the best peanuts available. Not to be outdone, my mother makes chocolate dipped coconut balls that would rival those of any candy maker. Both are pure decadence, but the few times a year when these treats are available, I refuse to miss out. Though they are the antithesis of health food, eating such treats on an occasional basis produces a significant amount of pleasure. Exceptions can be an important part of health and well-being, just as long as they are kept in proper perspective.

My "exceptions list" includes items such as ice cream, hamburger, pasta and bread, but I do not have them very often. As time goes on, it seems the list is getting shorter and I "need" these things less often. I also feel much better if I stay away from them. Keep an "exceptions list" for yourself and use it wisely.

When first changing to a healthy diet, you may find that many of your everyday foods are on the "exceptions list." In the beginning, at least for several months, it is probably best to "purge" your system completely and avoid them altogether. Gradually they can be added back on an occasional basis. When you get around to doing this, consider asking yourself questions such as: Is it something I really need right now? How much do I really want it? How bad will it make me feel if I do eat it? Can I get by with just a bite or two and still be happy?

Every now and then, life demands a special treat. Why waste it on some artificially-sweetened-processed-tofu thing, when what you really want is an ice cream sandwich? Go ahead and get the real thing, but possibly a smaller version of the real thing. And make it an exceptional treat to be savored on an occasional, not daily, basis.

CHAPTER 9

Daily Sustenance

The most challenging part of changing to a healthy diet is learning to like it. Children start with a very limited palate and gradually accept new foods as they are continually exposed to them. If, as an adult, you have never been exposed to different vegetables and other grains besides wheat, it is unlikely that you will have a taste for them. We could ship you off to an island where only these foods were available, but such drastic measures are really not necessary (though sometimes pleasant to consider!). You can create an island within your own world, just by defining better choices!

Anyone can learn to like a wide variety of foods if he or she makes the effort.

Start slowly. Begin to substitute brown rice, oats and other whole grains for wheat products. Gradually introduce different varieties of vegetables into your diet, with a target of half of daily food consumption coming from fresh vegetables. Use the Internet and the guidelines below to find ways to adapt your palate to vegetables and other foods. Use recipes that combine different healthy foods in one dish. Add small amounts of unfamiliar foods to a main course that you like very much, so that the taste is not overpowering. This is an especially good strategy for learning to like beans or certain vegetables. Before you know it, your tastes will change—I guarantee it.

When hunger strikes, most people will eat whatever is handy. Stock your pantry with only healthy food and the transition to a healthful diet will occur more rapidly!

CREATING A WELL-STOCKED KITCHEN

Menu plans are sometimes useful, but are more often limiting and frequently abandoned. Having a well-stocked kitchen and learning how to improvise offers a more functional approach. The focus of this section is stocking the kitchen with healthy food. Limiting availability to healthy foods is the first step in changing to a healthier diet!

The following lists offer examples for stocking the kitchen and pantry.

Basic condiments and spices

Spices, herbs, oils, and vinegars are a very important part of simple cooking. These ingredients allow the addition of flavor without added salt, sugar, and fat. Different combinations can completely change the style or taste of food.

Oils

There are many varieties of oils, each adding their own particular taste to food. Oils should be minimally refined and cold-pressed. Notice that corn oil is not on the list.

Olive oil	walnut oil	sesame oil
Canola oil	grapeseed oil (a spray can is handy)	
Macadamia nut oil		

Vinegar

Vinegar has a way of bringing out the flavor of food and can be used in many types of dishes. Different vinegars, of course, have different flavors.

Apple cider vinegar – an all-purpose vinegar.

Rice vinegar – a light vinegar for light cooking. Often used in Oriental dishes.

Malt vinegar – a tasty vinegar, great for seafood and potato dishes.

Balsamic vinegar – a robust vinegar made from red wine. Excellent for Italian dishes.

Fresh herbs

Fresh herbs are easy to grow in a simple garden from spring until fall and can also be grown indoors near a sunny window. Grocery stores often stock fresh herbs in the produce section. Though a selection of dried herbs is good to have on hand, choose fresh ones whenever you can.

Popular fresh herbs include basil, oregano, thyme, rosemary, marjoram, cilantro, dill, tarragon, fennel, and lemongrass.

Dry spices

Cinnamon, nutmeg, curry powder, cumin, chili powder, turmeric, Mexican oregano, saffron, allspice, garam masala, paprika, mustard powder, and cayenne pepper are must-haves. Add dried thyme, oregano, basil, and bay leaves when the fresh varieties are not available.

In the refrigerator: Low-sodium soy sauce, Worcestershire sauce, mild curry paste, a large jar of minced garlic, mustard, fresh ginger root or a jar of minced ginger, and hot chili sauce. There are various other bottled sauces that can make cooking simpler, but do not be afraid to make your own. And what refrigerator would be complete without a jar of pickle relish pushed to the far back corner?

Salad dressings and mayonnaise are now readily available with unrefined oil and better quality ingredients. Making your own salad dressing, however, is not very difficult, and recipes for every variety you can imagine can be found on the Internet.

Yogurt is a great snack food but is also useful in making creamy dressings and sauces. Choose organic plain (unsweetened) yogurt. Look for low-fat varieties. Strained or Greek yogurt (sometimes called yogurt cheese) is excellent, too.

Hummus is another multi-purpose food that you need to have on hand. Hummus is a tasty dip for vegetables, an alternative to mayonnaise as a spread for sandwiches, and a thickener for use in cooking. Garbanzo bean flour is a healthy substitute for corn starch or white flour when recipes call for a thickener. Nut butters (organic peanut, almond or sunflower) keep best in the refrigerator once opened and can also be used in cooking.

Refrigerator drawers should contain a seasonal assortment of fresh fruits and vegetables. Let the seasons and availability of local food dictate what's for dinner. Other staples include soymilk, almond milk or organic milk, soy milk, iced tea, orange juice, representative samples of cheese such as sharp cheddar, Swiss, and parmesan, free-range eggs, and a container of butter/canola oil blend. Dates, figs, prunes and other dried fruits are great snacks. Try tofu or tempeh. And make sure there is room for a watermelon during summer months.

In the freezer: The freezer is the place to store nuts, all kept in tight containers so they will not become freezer burned. Whole grain flours should be kept here, too, as well as free-range meats and flash-frozen salmon, shrimp and other seafood. Fresh-frozen organic berries and vegetables are often less expensive than fresh. Keep frozen bananas on hand as an ice cream substitute. Ice cream or ice cream substitutes (soy or coconut) for an occasional treat.

In the pantry: Basic suggestions for healthy items to have on hand include brown basmati rice, jasmine rice, wild rice, dried red and green lentils, barley, quinoa and canned items. A couple of cans of crushed organic tomatoes and a can of tomato paste are essential, along with canned beans such as red kidney, black beans, cannoli beans, navy beans and pinto beans. A small can of coconut milk is a necessity for Thai cooking. Also keep gluten-free crackers, organic corn chips and Durum wheat pasta on hand.

TIPS ON SHOPPING

The produce section should account for half of items in the grocery cart. The remainder of a typical shopping trip is devoted to replacing staples such as soymilk, yogurt, eggs, oatmeal, rice, canned or bottled goods and sometimes meat and cheese. Most items in the central part of the store and freezer sections are best left untouched. Pass the cereal and cookie aisles on by.

As a physician with a keen interest in nutrition, it's hard not to notice what other people have in their carts at the grocery store. I invariably make assumptions about their health risks. Sometimes I think I could do a better job assessing someone's health status by following them around in the grocery store than by doing a screening exam at the office. Maybe I could offer it as a way to save money in the new healthcare system. Instead of going to the office, I could be paid to hang around the grocery store and give nutritional advice.

It often surprises me that my cart full of fresh items is usually about the same price as the cartload of packaged goods that other people are willing to pay for. Packaging adds cost, and meat, especially, adds cost. People who buy packaged food often tend to buy a lot of meat. I like the flavor of meat as much as anyone else, but a little bit goes a long way. Our healthcare expenditures would immediately go down if everyone in the country started buying half as much meat and packaged foods as they are right now.

Food shopping needn't be limited to grocery stores. Local seafood markets, fruit and vegetable stands and farmers markets add new dimensions to food shopping. Buying from local markets and growers whenever you can is an important way to support your community. Trips to the state farmers' market with a large cooler are a special treat.

Mail order can be a practical way to obtain quality food at reasonable prices. Free-range meats of different varieties are available online. My freezer always contains a large package of mixed nuts obtained from a reputable source.

Remember to bring your own cloth bags on shopping trips!

STARTING THE DAY OFF RIGHT

On the path to a healthful diet, breakfast is a great starting point. This simple meal is often overlooked, but it may be the most important meal of the day. The energy provided by breakfast gives your body a jump start on the morning. It does not have to be complex or time-consuming, but also it does not have to be boring. Make note that your stomach may need some time to adjust if breakfast is not a part of your normal routine!

Start with familiar foods and gradually add variety. Carbohydrates and grain products can be part of a healthful breakfast, but products that cause "sugar-surges," such as bagels, donuts, pastries and the like, should be left behind—permanently. A grain-free breakfast is perfectly acceptable.

Beverages are an important part of breakfast. Strict coffee drinkers should try substituting hot tea (regular or green) occasionally. Fresh orange juice is great way to get a boost of Vitamin C and natural folates in the morning—the fruit sugar will be burned during the day.

Healthy ways to start your day
- **Veggies for breakfast!** Sauté chopped mushrooms in a non-stick pan with minced garlic. Mix in a handful of frozen chopped spinach. Allow the spinach to melt and cook. Beat an egg with a splash of soy milk and pour into the spinach-mushroom mix. Season with sea salt, pepper, a splash of soy sauce to add flavor and/or a sprinkle of parmesan cheese. Cook until the egg is done.

  Try other vegetables! Yellow squash, onion, and spinach with a handful of walnuts thrown in at the end works well!

- **Organic oatmeal (steel-cut or rolled whole oats)** with a drizzle of honey, raisins, cinnamon, soymilk (or almond milk), and a pat of butter is a great way to start the day. Do not stop with oatmeal. Most other whole grains can be used in this fashion as a hot breakfast cereal. Consider quinoa, barley or a mix of several different whole grains. A large pot of barley can be used in various ways for both main meals and breakfasts.

My 2-hour post-prandial (after eating) blood glucose level was consistently 90 or below after eating a bowl of steel-cut oats with honey, as compared to boxed cereals that typically resulted in blood glucose levels in the 140 range.

- **Homemade granola.** Store-bought varieties are always saturated with sugar and should be avoided. Making your own is so easy. Measure about 6 cups of rolled whole grain oats in a large bowl. (You can substitute barley for part of this, for variety.) Mix in a sprinkling of salt, ground nutmeg, cinnamon, ginger or allspice. Drizzle 4 tablespoons of canola oil and 1/3 cup of honey over the grain and mix. Spread onto a large baking tray and bake at 300°F for about 30 minutes, until golden brown. Stir every 10 minutes. During the last 10 minutes, add pumpkin seeds, sunflower seeds, coconut or chopped pecans. After the mixture comes out of the oven, cool and then add raisins, dried blueberries or other dried fruit. Store in a sealed container. This is good with yogurt, soymilk, almond milk, coconut milk, organic cow's milk or organic goat's milk.

- **Boxed cereals?** Virtually all boxed cereals are either saturated with sugar or processed wheat and <u>should</u> <u>be</u> <u>avoided</u>. Plain shredded wheat is the only boxed cereal that does not contain sugar, but with wheat as a primary ingredient, this product should be avoided by wheat sensitive individuals (a large portion of the population). For individuals who tolerate wheat, shredded wheat can be added as an *occasional* breakfast item.

The big yellow box with little round oat cereal is a better option than most, but finely ground oat flour still releases glucose faster than whole grain oats and the product still contains refined sugar, corn starch and wheat starch.

- **Fresh fruit and yogurt.** Opt for plain, unsweetened yogurt with fresh fruit and/or some type of sweetener such as a bit of agave honey, Stevia or Xylitol. Granola, pumpkin seeds, pecans, flax meal, or chia seeds can be added to the yogurt for texture. Making your own yogurt saves money and is easier than you think. Yogurt makers are available at most department stores and online.

- **Brown rice for breakfast.** Whenever rice is part of a meal, cook extra for use in other meals. Leftover brown rice is perfect for breakfast. Rice, warmed with raisins, walnuts, butter and soymilk makes for a soothing breakfast on a cold day. Taking it in another direction, rice can be mixed with leftover vegetables and crumbles of soy sausage.

- **Eggs are fine several times a week** (unless you have a hereditary cholesterol problem). Hard-boiled, poached, fried, or scrambled, eggs take very little time. Leave off the toast for a change, and try a side of plantains sautéed in butter or coconut oil or black beans with salsa. The possibilities are almost unlimited!

   Fried eggs should be cooked on low heat.

- **Something other than toast.** Leftover sweet potato is perfect for breakfast. Whenever having sweet potatoes for supper, pull one out of the oven before it is quite done and save it in the refrigerator. The next morning, slice the potato into half-inch thick slices, remove the peel and pan-fry lightly to heat. Sliced sweet potatoes can be cooked alongside eggs. Sweet potatoes can also be cubed and cooked like "hash browns."

- **Fresh fruit on the side.** Consider a mix of melon, bananas, blueberries, raspberries, strawberries, grapefruit, oranges, or other fruits. The sugars will be burned as the day goes on.

- **Frijoles in the morning.** Beans for breakfast? Absolutely! Scrambled eggs with salsa and seasoned black beans on the side make an excellent breakfast. Add plantains or bananas sautéed in macadamia nut oil with cinnamon and you have really gone south of the border!

- **Waffles.** Waffles freeze quite well and make a perfect on-the-go breakfast. Gluten-free waffles are available, but the best waffles are the ones made from scratch. Thaw in the microwave for a few seconds, pop them in the toaster, and they taste even better than right off the waffle iron.

On weekends, I frequently make whole grain waffles from scratch and freeze extras for use during the week (see recipe below under weekend breakfasts).

- **Poached eggs, sprouted-grain toast and quinoa with butter.** Quinoa is very good for breakfast and is reminiscent of corn grits. It can also be served like oatmeal with milk, butter, brown sugar and raisins. Sprouted grain bread is lower in carbohydrate than other whole grain breads, but still contains gluten.

- **Healthier hash browns.** Potatoes with less starch, such as the little red ones, are okay for occasional eating. Start with pre-cooked potatoes (a good way to use leftovers). Chop up an onion and a bell pepper. Use an amount equal in volume to that of the potatoes. Cut the potatoes into cubes or small slices. Sauté the potatoes, onions, peppers in olive oil on medium-high heat until brown. Add salt and red pepper to taste. Serve with a fried egg. This recipe is also quite good using sweet potatoes (avoid overcooking potatoes prior to use in the sauté) or even left-over rutabagas.

- **Smoothie.** See Small Meals in the next section for a meal-substitute smoothie. Smoothies can be made ahead of time for healthy on-the-go meals.

WEEKEND BREAKFASTS (also make great light evening meals)
- **Wheat-free waffles.** Get your waffle iron ready! Virtually any grain can be used, and the recipe can vary depending on the types of grains on hand.

I have made this recipe with the addition of coconut flour and also teff flour (a very small kernel grain from Africa).

¾ cup whole grain buckwheat flour
¾ cup whole grain oat flour
½ cup pecans or walnuts, ground in a food processor
1 tsp. baking powder
3 T. canola oil
1 egg
½ can of organic pumpkin or sweet potatoes

1 cup soy or almond milk (more or less, to achieve a pourable batter)

Cook as per directions with your waffle iron. Top with pure maple syrup or fruit and yogurt. For a side item, try soy sausage.

My 2-hour postprandial blood glucose after one of these waffles—89!

- **Veggie omelet.** Here's how to make a perfect omelet. By hand, beat 4 to 6 eggs with salt, pepper, and a splash of soymilk. Season a 10-inch, rounded edge sautéed pan with non-stick cooking spray (eggs are a challenge to cook without a non-stick pan). Pour the egg mixture into the cold pan about a quarter inch deep. **Starting with a cold pan is an important key to success!** Place the pan on the stove with low-medium heat. Sprinkle fresh grated parmesan cheese on top. The omelet is done when there is no liquid on top and the cheese is melted. While the omelet is cooking, sautéed chopped onions, mushrooms, peppers, spinach, tomatoes, garlic, and fresh oregano in olive oil. Spread this mixture on top of the omelet and fold with two spatulas. Generally, this is a meal in itself, but it can be garnished with fruit or soy sausage.

- **Salmon patties and sprouted-grain toast.** In many cultures, fish is a breakfast staple. For the patties, mix leftover grilled salmon or canned wild salmon with an egg, chopped onion, chopped bell peppers, garlic, salt, pepper, and oat flour. Form into patties and cook in a frying pan seasoned with non-stick spray. Cook until brown and serve with sprouted-grain toast.

HEALTHY FOOD ON THE GO

Here in America we tend to eat lightly during the day and save our big meal for the end of the day. Many experts would suggest that the European plan of eating a main meal in the middle of the day and eating lightly in the evening is a healthier alternative. No doubt, this style of eating is better for digestion and probably less conducive to weight gain, but fitting a large meal into the middle of an American day is a real challenge—avoiding a big meal altogether may be a possible solution. Eating small amounts throughout the day prevents and suppresses the urge to eat large amounts. On some days, consider having several substantial snacks during the day and then a lighter meal at night. Eating lunch instead of dinner at a nice sit-down restaurant is pleasant way to break up the day. Midday meals at better restaurants tend to be lighter and healthier.

For on-the-go days there are many options to choose from without resorting to typical fast-food fare.

SMALL AND EXTRA-QUICK MEALS

Some of the most pleasant meals I can remember in my lifetime have been the simple ones. A favorite pastime for my family has been hiking in various different national parks around the country. Day hikes usually include a simple meal along the way. Standard fare includes carrots and celery with hummus, gluten-free crackers with nut-butter, Swiss cheese, apples, berries, chocolate, and bottles of water. Any preparation is done with a pocket knife and the "table" is usually a rock overlooking some gorgeous valley, waterfall, or equally magnificent scene miles away from civilization. Food cannot taste any better than after you have walked half a day to end up in such a special place. These simple meals have become the most celebrated of our lives.

Simple meals can be some of the best because they do not require much preparation or cleanup. They can be fixed anytime during the day or evening. A wide assortment of such meals is possible. Though some of the items mentioned below may seem foreign to your taste buds, change can happen over time.

My office staff constantly makes fun of my lunches. I think nothing of microwaving a collection of cabbage and mushrooms seasoned with olive oil and ginger and eaten with a can of herring or sardines. It's all a matter of what you get used to. Sometimes good health is worth a little compromise.

Vegetable bowls. Fresh vegetables, the most important of our food sources, are often left off the menu completely. Even those who like vegetables sometimes find it hard to consume a full quota each day.

A concept I call "vegetable bowls" is a possible solution. At the office, I keep a selection of fresh and frozen vegetables in the refrigerator at all times. It takes about five minutes to fill a bowl with a varying assortment of different chopped vegetables. The only tools necessary are a large (3-4 cup) glass bowl with a lid, a cutting board, a large knife and a spoon. Five minutes in the microwave and you have a bowl of fresh steamed vegetables.

The key to making vegetables palatable is the addition of spices and a little bit of fat. Having variety of bottled sauces, pesto and spices on hand along with a bottle of olive oil completes the ingredients list. Brown rice, chicken or shrimp brought in from home also make flavorful additions. This concept can also be prepared at home the night before and microwaved at lunch the next day. Below are some suggestions for items and possible seasoning combinations:

Vegetables   carrots, cabbage, peppers, celery, edamame (fresh soybeans), broccoli, fresh green beans, zucchini, onion, and peas.

Other items   kidney beans, black beans, lentils, black-eyed peas, hummus, brown rice, pre-cooked chicken, pre-cooked shrimp. Dried fruit, such as prunes, can add sweetness and flavor. Walnuts, added at the end, provide healthy fats and crunch.

Seasonings   *Italian:*   green pesto or sun-dried tomato pesto, garlic, parmesan. *Oriental:* ginger, garlic, soy sauce. *Indian:* ginger, garlic, curry paste. Olive oil can be added to a dish for extra flavor.

Try it. Add a vegetable bowl to your routine at least several times a week. There are almost an infinite number of possible combinations. From a health perspective, it will never be rivaled by something out of a bag or package, in quality or taste. When you first start out, stick with items that seem familiar, and then gradually expand your tastes. Do not be afraid to think outside the box. Vegetable bowls can also be done as a light stir-fry and served with brown basmati rice.

Other suggestions for quick meals during the day or in the evening:

- **Leftovers!** Some of the best and quickest lunches are leftovers. The night before, cook extra for the evening meal with the intention of allowing for lunch the next day. Often extras from one meal can also provide the raw ingredients for subsequent meals. You just have to get into the habit of thinking ahead when cooking a meal.

- **Soup.** Soups are so easy to make and can be frozen for later use. During winter months, a large pot of soup made on the weekend can provide a couple of evening meals and several lunches. Avoid canned soups (except for those containing mainly beans or lentils, which tend to retain their nutritional value when canned). Because of the amount of heat required for canning soups, the nutritional value of most vegetables is lost in processing.

  Recently, a soup company came out with a campaign advertising "0" calories and "0" fat. What they did not advertise was "0" nutrition.

- **Mixed greens salad.** Search for fresh organic lettuces. Organic spinach is also available. The deeper the green, the more substantial the nutritional value. Iceberg lettuce has virtually no nutritional value and should be avoided. With choices like fresh cut vegetables, boiled egg, crumbled walnuts, pumpkin seeds, avocado, grapes, blueberries, raisins, chopped red bell peppers, carrots, canned wild salmon, and/or tofu, there are almost unlimited salad toppings.

- **Sandwiches.** Sandwiches are the quintessential on-the-go American food—and despite the standard presence of bread, sandwiches can be made into healthy choices. Thin-sliced, sprouted-grain bread or gluten-free bread are healthful choices, but it actually doesn't have to be bread at all. Two romaine lettuce leaves will suffice. Take a break from the classic meat and cheese by substituting tomatoes, cucumbers, avocado, shredded carrots, leftover grilled vegetables or sautéed portabella mushrooms into your sandwich. Hummus is a great spread with vegetables. A little bit of olive oil and vinegar also works wonderfully well.

- **Beans and rice.** Whenever you cook rice, cook extra. Beans can be used to change the flavor of the dish. Spice it up with the addition of stir-fried vegetables, fresh minced herbs and garlic, Mexican spices like cumin and chili powder, seafood, or chicken. This same idea can be used with other grains such as barley or quinoa.

- **Leftover quinoa.** Mix with a spoonful of red pepper hummus and crushed organic tomatoes, and microwave for a minute. The combination is surprisingly tasty. As a side, add a simple slaw made with shredded cabbage and carrots, diced apples, raisins, a bit of mayonnaise (try the olive oil variety), a little mustard, salt, pepper, paprika, and you have a nutritious meal.

- **Tofu** with ginger dressing, baked in a toaster oven for 20 minutes. To most people tofu, by itself, is bland and relatively tasteless, but tofu soaks up any flavor added to it. If cooked properly, tofu can be a tasteful food source. Serve this dish with steamed cabbage.

  The people of Okinawa, Japan enjoy very high soy consumption and can boast of very low rates of breast and prostate cancer. This, alone, is reason enough to consider adapting to the taste of tofu. Look for organic, non-GMO varieties.

- **Steamed fresh salmon** with ginger sauce along with steamed edamame, mushrooms, and soy sauce. Edamame is the Japanese name for fresh soybeans. The taste is somewhere between a pea and a butterbean.

- **ALT.** Avocado, lettuce and tomato on whole sprouted-grain bread. The fat in avocado has a flavor that substitutes well for bacon, making for a healthy and flavorful alternative to a BLT.

- **Sautéed chicken breast.** Sauté free-range organic chicken breast in olive on low heat. After the meat is seared, add mushrooms, a splash of white wine, capers and salt and pepper. Cover and cook on low until the meat is cooked through. Sprinkle parmesan cheese on top and serve with steamed broccoli or asparagus.

- **A taste of the ocean.** Seaweed is a foreign taste to most westerners, but becomes quite acceptable when blended with other vegetables. For this dish, sauté chopped onions, shitake mushrooms, shredded cabbage and thin-sliced zucchini squash in canola oil on low heat until tender. Heat 2 teaspoons dried wachame seaweed in water with 1 teaspoon of miso paste in the microwave. Seaweed hydrates quickly. Miso is made from soybeans and tastes similar to soy sauce. After the seaweed and miso are hydrated, blend into the vegetable mixture. Fresh shrimp, chicken, or a couple of beaten eggs can be added for a protein source. This nutritious meal can be served any time of day, including breakfast!

- **Pick-me-up smorgasbord.** A meal does not always have to be well-defined. Get creative! Sometimes an assortment makes quite an adequate meal.

- **Smoothie, 8 oz.** per serving
  1-2 teaspoons organic virgin coconut oil
  2 tablespoons chia seeds
  1 scoop protein powder (egg white, whey, rice, fermented soy, or hemp)
  Soy milk and/or plain yogurt
  Berries (blueberries, blackberries, strawberries, raspberries, or any other)—fresh or frozen

  Optional ingredients:
  Ice
  Carrot
  Celery
  Greens – kale, Romaine lettuce, spinach
  Canned pumpkin or sweet potatoes (great with peaches)
  Coconut
  Banana
  Soft tofu
  Peanut butter
  Powdered greens mix
  Cocoa powder

  Mix ingredients and blend thoroughly in a blender.

SNACKS AND HUNGER BUSTERS

Snacking during the day is important. Snacking provides a break from the everyday grind and helps stop hunger in its tracks. Ravenous hunger can lead to eating too fast and over-eating at mealtimes. The types of snack foods, however, are extremely important.

For many individuals, being overweight is directly related to eating the wrong types of snack foods!

Typical snack foods are a processed-food nightmare. You know the types – cakes, cookies, donuts, potato chips, etc. They generally have all three of the most concerning ingredients of processed food–rapid-glucose-releasing carbs, hydrogenated oils, and lots of fructose. Remember, fructose drives appetite instead of suppressing it! Purging snack foods containing these ingredients actually reduces intensity of hunger and curbs excessive snacking.

Processed snack foods should be avoided. Even the ones labeled as "health foods" contain sugar (sugar is sugar, organic or not) and fats that are often rancid.

- Cut vegetables—carrots, celery, yellow squash, cucumbers—dipped in hummus are a low- calorie mainstay snack.

  Celery contains important cancer-fighting chemicals, can lower blood pressure in hypertensive individuals and is natural way to help normalize low testosterone levels in men. Several stalks a day are recommended. Carrots contain carotenoids, chemicals that protect eyes and skin. Eat a few carrots each day.

- Sliced organic apple with nut butter (sunflower, peanut, cashew, or almond) is a satisfying snack.

- Low-carb crackers (Wasa brand or other <12 gram carbohydrate cracker) or gluten-free seed crackers, lightly spread with nut butter, hummus or a piece of cheese.

  Spinach-artichoke spread: blend a can of artichokes with an equal amount of chopped spinach (fresh leaves can be used) in a food processor. Blend in 1-2 tablespoons of mayonnaise, 1 tablespoon of shredded parmesan cheese, ½ squeezed lemon, salt and pepper. Pine nuts, 1 tablespoon, can be added for flavor.

- One half of a ripe avocado with salt and pepper is an adequate snack by itself. You can add a few whole-grain organic corn chips.

  Avocados are a very healthy snack food, but finding a perfectly ripe avocado that has not been bruised in the store is tricky. To get the best ones, choose avocados that are firm and green, but just starting to turn black. Store on the counter (not on the refrigerator) so they will continue to ripen. Slight softening and a shift toward black usually confirms a ripe avocado. Slice in half lengthwise and remove the seed. The contents can be scooped out with a spoon.

- Roll-ups. A slice of organic turkey wrapped in a slice of Swiss cheese is an excellent low-carb snack.

- A handful of fresh pumpkin seeds with a piece of crystalized ginger is very satisfying. Pumpkin seeds may reduce prostate disease.

- Lettuce wraps. Try finely chopped nuts, roasted chicken or canned salmon, grated carrots, chopped celery and green onion wrapped in romaine lettuce.

- Whole fruit is a perfect snack food, but should be kept in the context of a snack and not a meal. Apples, oranges, cherries, pears, bananas, plums, melons, and berries of any type are a great way to fill the hunger void. Dried fruit such as prunes, raisins, apricots, and dates are adequate substitutes when fresh is not available. Please note, however, that fruit should be used in strict moderation if weight loss is the goal.

  Bananas never go bad around my house. As soon as they ripen, whole bananas are peeled, halved, wrapped in plastic wrap or waxed paper and placed in the freezer for a treat that is nearly equal to ice cream. Shave on dark chocolate for an extra special indulgence.

- If you have a juicer, fruit and vegetable juices make refreshing, healthy treats. Try a combination of carrots, fresh ginger, celery, romaine lettuce and an apple. Fresh berries and citrus are a tasty combination. The possibilities are unlimited.

- Whole grain organic corn chips (in moderation) with hummus or salsa.

- Nuts in general make great snacks. A snack mix can be made with almonds, pecans, Brazil nuts, cashews, walnuts, sunflower seeds, pumpkin seeds, raisins, and carob or chocolate chips. This keeps very well in the freezer. Nuts are high in fat, but the fats are healthy. You could gain weight if you ate enough of them, but a handful or two a day should not be a problem with regular exercise.

A handful of fresh pecans with dark chocolate chips beats any snack bar for health and taste!

- Try plain organic yogurt sweetened with vanilla stevia and topped with ground chia seeds or flaxseed, berries, pecans or walnuts.

  The very best yogurt is homemade. Yogurt makers are inexpensive and the process is very simple. Homemade yogurt costs a fraction of the store-bought version.

- A "smoothie" takes no time at all. Toss several different types of frozen berries or fruit into a blender. Add a scoop of low-fat yogurt along with a squirt of fresh flaxseed oil and a package of Stevia or a little honey as a sweetener. Pour in enough soymilk to cover everything. Blend until the contents are smooth and pour an extremely refreshing and healthy snack.

- Organic popcorn is a satisfactory snack, especially if you stay away from the processed and packaged varieties. For as long as I can remember we have had used a device called a "Whirley Pop" (www.popcornpopper.com) popcorn popper that agitates the kernels of corn as they are being heated on the stove. One teaspoon of macadamia nut oil, a pat of butter, a little salt and you will have the best tasting popcorn on earth.

- Don't forget snack foods that aren't typical snack foods. There is nothing wrong with eating leftovers. Most leftovers are much lower in calories than average snack foods.

- A cup of hot tea can, by itself, be an adequate appetite suppressant.

The style of snacking is dependent on the activity level of the day. At the office, low energy nibbles are preferred, whereas a five mile hike in the mountains would dictate the need for high energy snacks such as chocolate or peanut butter. Through-hikers on the Appalachian Trail actually eat large amounts of peanut butter just to maintain weight.

FULL MEALS

In an ideal world, the largest meal would occur in the middle of the day and be followed by an afternoon siesta. While this luxury is commonly observed during holidays, most people find it impractical for everyday life. In America, a light midday meal is typically followed by a full meal at the end of the day. For working adults with busy lifestyles, cooking that meal can be a real inconvenience. It should not be. Meals prepared from fresh ingredients are always healthier than those prepared in a restaurant or by a food factory.

Achieving optimal health requires knowing how to prepare food simply and easily from whatever is on hand. In the following section, naivety about cooking is assumed and the start is from ground zero. The series of meals are simple enough for any novice to handle, but anyone should find tasty. Try several different ones each week. From here you should be able to go "solo" and move on to ideas of your own without being encumbered by a recipe book.

With a minimal investment of time and effort, anyone should be able to retrieve items already on hand from the refrigerator and pantry and construct a tasty and healthy meal—the art of simple cooking. Whether for a single individual or a whole family, this goal can even be accomplished even after a long day at work.

When choosing items for a meal, start with the most perishable produce first. This practice, in itself, can be a guide to meal planning. Check the refrigerator vegetable bin frequently—don't allow your valuable produce to become a compost pile!

Add other items to round out the meal. Take advantage of "batch" items. If rice is on the menu, cook enough to make several different dishes during the week. The same goes for steamed vegetables. A week's worth of different meals can be constructed using precooked vegetables with different spices, sauces, and added meats.

Preferential tastes for sugar and fat can be respected, without becoming a slave to them. A bit of dried fruit or fruit jam, a drizzle of honey or a handful of nuts accentuates the flavor of food without robbing health benefits. Herbs and spices enliven any food!

BASIC STIR-FRY

Have you ever been to a Mongolian barbeque? Fresh raw foods, including a variety of vegetables, meats, seafood and seasonings, are displayed for customers in salad bar-like fashion. Each person files through a line and fill bowls with preferential choices. The bowl of ingredients is presented to a cook, who runs them around a large flat grill and hands back a plate of piping-hot, fresh food of the customer's own creation. The whole process takes about five minutes and ten different people could go through the line and come out with ten different meals. This is the essence of simple cooking: fast, easy, and with endless variations.

Following the lead of the Mongolian barbeque, a simple stir-fry can be used to achieve the same goal. Any large, stainless steel, flat-bottomed pan (10-12 inches in diameter) will do. A reasonable quality stainless pan can be purchased at a discount store without having to fork over an entire paycheck. Add a large rounded knife for cutting vegetables and mincing herbs, a thin knife for trimming meat, a cutting board, a big spoon and a covered pan to cook rice in and you have the makings of a basic kitchen. Throw in a large soup pot, a vegetable steamer, and an outdoor grill and you are set for a full range of cooking! For pots and pans I generally recommend using steel and staying away from aluminum and non-stick coated cookware (except for cooking eggs—nearly impossible to clean without non-stick).

The ingredients

What goes into this meal depends on your personal tastes. Start with things that you genuinely like. Cooking two versions is easy—adults and children often have different tastes. The whole family can join in: Children and husbands should be comfortable in the kitchen and know how to cook!

When my kids were younger, I would stir-fry the meat first with seasonings and set it aside. Then I would stir-fry vegetables for my wife and me and add some of the meat mixture in for flavor. Adapting to the taste of vegetables takes time for some individuals. As time went on I would mince small amounts of a certain vegetable into the kids' version until they became used to it. Eventually, only one version was necessary for all of us.

The meal we are about to cook blends flavors to come up with a unique taste. Different vegetables, oils, meats, and seasonings all affect the flavor of a dish. The amount of variety possible is almost infinite. Healthy foods can be added gradually as taste adapts. Broccoli may not be your favorite, but instead of being ignored altogether, it can be incorporated into a blend with other flavors. Even the pickiest individuals should be able to mix up a list of ingredients that they can enjoy.

Pick your favorites and then add smaller amounts of others that are less familiar. The foreign flavors will be less noticeable.

Vegetables

broccoli	cabbage	carrots	green peas
cauliflower	zucchini	onions	snow peas
eggplant	spinach	asparagus	spring onions
bok choy	celery	mushrooms	yellow squash
spring onions		green beans	
edamame (soybeans)		bell pepper (red, green, yellow)	

Meats

chicken	shrimp	scallops	squid
fish	pork	beef	crab

Other Ingredients

prunes (add sweetness)
sesame seeds
beans (black, white or red)
tofu or tempeh
nuts (walnuts, cashews, or sliced almonds)

Basic seasonings for a Chinese style stir fry

canola oil (heat tolerant)

(olive or macadamia nut oil is fine if care is taken not to overheat the oil)

soy sauce (low salt)	vegetable or chicken broth
minced garlic	fresh grated ginger
fresh minced cilantro	fresh minced basil

Generally this dish is accompanied by rice, but rice can be omitted to reduce carbohydrates. Brown basmati rice is preferred for fiber, flavor, protein-content, and paucity of starch.

The rice is the first thing to go on the stove. Brown basmati rice takes about 45 minutes to prepare. Next is preparation of raw materials—vegetables are chopped, meats are sliced, and herbs are minced. A two-quart pitcher of chopped ingredients is generally more than enough for four people, but do not be afraid to cook extra, since leftovers make nutritious lunches.

Chopping vegetables and slicing meat

A good quality, wide blade knife with a rounded bottom across the edge is preferred for chopping vegetables. Note that good does not necessarily mean expensive. Any type of cutting board will do, but bamboo holds up quite well.

Meat generally requires a sharp thin-blade knife. If using chicken, remove the skin. If using beef (or pork), trim any fat. Slice the meat into quarter- to half- inch strips. Use a plastic cutting board for meat to avoid bacterial build-up.

Fresh herbs

Fresh herbs are widely available and have much more flavor than their dried counterparts. Lay a handful of herbs on a wooden cutting board. Grasp the top of a large rounded-blade knife with both hands. Chop across the herbs with a rapid chopping motion. After one pass, use the edge of the blade to pull the pile into a row. Chop across the row. Repeat until the herbs are finely minced.

Homemade teriyaki sauce

Mix ¼-½ cup of low salt soy sauce with a cup of organic chicken or vegetable broth. Add a teaspoon of rice wine vinegar. Grate in a tbsp. of fresh ginger. Add a tsp. of fresh garlic and a tsp. of brown sugar. This a great sauce for many dishes and as a marinade for grilling.

Low-heat stir-fry

Traditional stir-frying is done over high heat with a wok, but burning the oil is absolutely unavoidable. While this is a popular method of cooking, gradually I have moved toward a low heat stir-fry. The method is easier, tastes better and is even healthier. It is actually closer to steaming, but retains the flavor of stir-fry. A 10-12 inch stainless sauté pan has replaced a wok as my favorite pan. Heat the pan on low to low-medium heat. When hot, pour in about a three inch circle of oil. Place onions and mushrooms in first and cook with the pan covered until tender. Stir enough to prevent burning. Add all other ingredients including seasonings and stir to coat with oil. Add 1-2 tablespoons of vegetable broth and cover. Simmer about five to ten extra minutes until vegetables are tender and meat is cooked. Nuts or seeds go in last.

Shift the ingredients and change the spices and you have a completely different flavor. Once you have the basic concept down, try several of the following low-heat stir-fry options.

Southeast Asian stir-fry

Any vegetables from the list will work, but milder flavored vegetables such as snow peas or spring onions are the best choices. Meat can include chicken, shrimp, or no meat at all! Extra-firm tofu concentrates all the flavors in the dish, and makes for a pleasant addition. Minced herbs can include either basil or cilantro. Lemongrass is also an excellent choice.

Jasmine rice is a fragrant, light rice that goes especially well with Thai or Indian cooking. It only takes about 15 minutes to prepare.

The many flavors found in this sauce define the essence of Thai cooking. Combine 1 cup vegetable or chicken broth, ¼ cup low sodium soy sauce, 2 tablespoons minced fresh ginger, ½-1 cup light coconut milk, 1 teaspoon brown sugar, ½ teaspoon red chili sauce, ½-1 teaspoon mild curry paste, ½ lime (squeezed), 1-2 teaspoons of rice wine vinegar, and 1 teaspoon minced garlic. Peanuts and peanut butter within the sauce make delicious variations of Thai.

Cook and serve this dish in exactly the same manner as the previous one.

Middle-eastern stir-fry

The same vegetables can be used as previous dishes, but again the sauce provides a completely different twist. It can be centered on chicken, tofu, or prepared as a totally vegetarian meal. For something different, serve over red lentils.

A little prep work is required for the sauce. Start with a small to medium onion and a red bell pepper, chopped and sautéed in olive oil. Add 1-2 teaspoons of minced garlic. Stir in one can of crushed organic tomatoes or tomato sauce.

Now for the spices: 1 tablespoon of chili powder, 1 teaspoon of ginger powder, 1 teaspoon of ground cumin, 1 teaspoon of ground turmeric, 1 tablespoon of mild curry paste, a half teaspoon of red chili sauce or minced red chili (cayenne), a pinch of sugar, and salt to taste.

Cook this dish in the same fashion as the previous ones. Mix in enough sauce to cover the vegetables. Save the unused sauce. This spicy tomato sauce can be used in a variety of dishes.

Pasta Primavera

Next we move to an Italian-style pasta dish. Vegetables that work well include zucchini, onion, mushrooms, bell pepper, and carrots. Shrimp are especially good in this one. The "sauce" is not made separately, but is created as you go.

Prepare the vegetables as per low-heat stir-fry instructions. Add 1 teaspoon of minced garlic. Add a whole handful of minced fresh basil and oregano (dried herbs will do in a pinch). Other seasoning additions can include pine nuts and chili powder.

Next, add 2 cups of fresh cherry tomatoes or 1 can crushed tomatoes. For extra flavor, stir in a couple of teaspoons of balsamic vinegar. Simmer until the tomatoes are broken apart and mixed in (you can help them with the back of a spoon if you like). Add salt to taste. Stir in 2 tablespoonful's of strained yogurt (Greek yogurt) and sprinkle freshly shredded parmesan cheese on top.

> *Pasta primavera would be seemingly incomplete without pasta, but for individuals trying to lose weight or avoiding grains, this dish is perfectly acceptable without it. Even with pasta, this should be a predominantly vegetable meal. Contrast this to the mountain of pasta consumed on an almost daily basis by many Americans!*

> *Wheat pasta is typically made from durum wheat; a different wheat species than that used to make bread and baked goods. Pasta made from durum wheat does not raise blood glucose levels nearly as fast as baked goods. When proportionally outweighed by vegetables and meat, pasta is an acceptable (though occasional) addition to a healthful diet—unless, of course, gluten sensitivity is suspected. Whole-grain pasta does not offer additional health benefits; oddly, it seems to raise blood glucose as fast or faster than the plain variety.*

> *A company called Dreamfields (www.dreamfields-foods.com) has created pasta with a low glycemic index (low potential for releasing glucose). The addition of non-digestible fiber slows absorption of glucose. Interestingly, the type of fiber added also feeds favorable bacteria in the intestinal tract. This is the type of innovation that we like to see from the food industry!*

How to make perfect pasta

Pour one to two quarts of water (depending on the amount of pasta) into a pot and bring to a boil. Add salt to taste. Add a tsp. of olive oil to prevent sticking. Add the pasta. Stir often, removing a piece now and then to see if it is ready. *Al dente* ("to the tooth") refers to pasta that has been cooked just enough to lose its crunchiness. At this point pour into a strainer to stop the cooking process.

Fish fajitas

Fish is the star ingredient for this quick and simple stir-fry, but vegetables are the supporting cast. Use any firm-textured fish such as triggerfish, grouper or Mahi-Mahi. Any of the vegetables from the previous list will work, but onions, bell peppers, shredded cabbage, and sometimes zucchini or mushrooms seem to fit best. How much of each ingredient depends on your taste. Again, the spices make the dish.

Sauté the vegetables over low heat as per previous directions. Add as much garlic as you like and a handful of minced cilantro. Spiciness and heat can be added with minced hot red pepper. Usually one small pepper with the seeds removed is plenty. The seeds account for much of the "heat" of the pepper. Mince very finely. Be careful about touching your face or eyes if you handle the pepper. Red chili sauce is an adequate substitute. When the vegetables begin to soften, add the fish (cut into chunks). Stir in 1-2 tablespoons of chili powder. Add ½ to 1 can of organic black beans.

This mixture can be served over shredded lettuce (or shredded cabbage) and tomatoes as a salad, or wrapped inside a soft tortilla. Toppings can include fresh salsa, shredded cheese, sour cream, guacamole, or avocado. Chicken works as well.

Easy Shrimp Creole

Traditionally the vegetables for this dish include tomatoes, onions, bell peppers, and celery, but consider adding other options such as zucchini and okra. Depending on the crowd, plan on about ¼ pound of peeled shrimp per person. Usually about one onion, one bell pepper (green, red, or yellow), 2 stalks or celery, and a large can of crushed tomatoes along with 1-2 lbs. of shrimp will do for four people. You can stretch this recipe with extra vegetables.

The spices include 1-2 teaspoons of cumin, 1-2 teaspoons of minced garlic, one minced cayenne pepper without seeds (unless you want it hot!) and 2 bay leafs.

Prepare the vegetables as per low-heat stir-fry instructions. Add the spices and the shrimp. Simmer until the shrimp are completely pink, stirring as needed. The tomatoes will generally add enough liquid. Serve over a bed of brown basmati rice.

Beef Stroganoff

For those who want a traditional meat version, use a lean cut of beef such as sirloin (free-range always preferred) cut into thin strips. The meat in this recipe can easily be replaced by either a medley of mushrooms or tempeh. The vegetables include onion, celery, mushrooms and tomatoes but many other vegetables such as eggplant can complement the flavor of this dish.

Stir-fry the meat first in a small amount of oil over low heat. When the meat browns, drain off the fat and add vegetables and seasonings. When the vegetables are tender, add a can of crushed tomatoes or a couple of chopped tomatoes. Water can be added if needed.

The seasonings for this dish include a handful of minced fresh oregano, a tablespoon of Worcestershire sauce, a small can of tomato paste, a teaspoon of garlic and a splash of balsamic vinegar. Stir in the seasonings at the same time as the tomatoes, and simmer covered for about 10 minutes. Remove from heat and stir in a couple of spoonful's of Greek yogurt. (Avoid adding the yogurt too early to prevent curdling.) This is a meal by itself, but it can be served with noodles—try buckwheat noodles (Japanese soba) for a change!

Wild rice and mushrooms

This next selection uses many of the same ingredients and spices as other dishes, but the flavor is completely altered by the presence of wild rice. Wild rice is prepared in the same way as brown rice and takes about the same amount of time. Start the rice ahead so that it can be cooking while preparing the main part of the dish.

Ideally, choose several different types of fresh mushrooms, chopped or sliced. Other vegetables can include chopped onion and red bell pepper, but try vegetables not used in other recipes. If you desire meat, the selection could include chicken, shrimp, or crab. Sauté the vegetables and meat over low heat in olive oil with seasonings including garlic, freshly minced thyme, freshly minced cilantro, and salt to taste. Rosemary also goes well.

Allow cooked mixture to cool slightly and then stir in 2-3 tablespoons of plain or Greek yogurt, 1-2 tablespoons of freshly grated Parmesan cheese, and 3-4 tablespoons of garbanzo bean paste or plain hummus. (Garbanzo bean flour can be found at most health food stores, some groceries and at www.bobsredmill.com.)

After all of these ingredients are mixed together, mix in several large spoonfuls of wild rice. The taste will be completely different from any of the dishes above.

Indian Curry

The essence of Indian cooking is the characteristic flavor of curry. Curry is actually not one spice, but a blend of many spices. Though the spices that make up curries are highly variable, most typical curries from India and the surrounding regions contain turmeric, coriander and cumin. Hot peppers are often added for spiciness. Curry can be found in dry form at the spice aisle and in wet form at the international foods sections of most grocery stores. Patak's Mild Curry Paste is a favorite that appeals to most people.

Preferred vegetables for this dish include cauliflower, onions, red potatoes, mushrooms, green peas, carrots and any types of squash. Chicken, any seafood or tofu are the meat choices. Any cooking oil can be used, but sesame oil is favored. The dish is prepared the same as all others. Add 1-2 teaspoons of curry paste as the vegetables are being cooked. Additional spices include garlic, fresh minced basil, ginger and pepper. Salt to taste. When the vegetables are tender, stir in 1-2 tablespoonful's of yogurt and 1-2 tablespoonful's of plain hummus.

Instead of rice, try this dish with green lentils. Prepare the lentils as per directions on the package and stir several large spoonful's into the dish.

In India, this dish would be made with ghee. Ghee is butter with the milk solids removed—almost pure saturated fat. Though the favor is rich, ghee is very heavy and would not win high marks for healthfulness. Ghee can be found in specialty groceries. If you would like to experience the flavor, add a small amount, in addition to normal cooking oil.

When following the concepts of simple cooking, do not fret about missing or unavailable ingredients. Improvisation is the byword. These dishes will all taste just fine with one or two of the recommended ingredients missing, or if a spice or ingredient does not suit your taste buds, leave it out!

Now that you have the basic concept, experiment. For inspiration, pick up a cooking magazine following the lighter side of cooking. Do internet searches for recipes using specific ingredients. Adapt the recipes to suit your particular tastes.

For weight loss considerations, note that any of the above dishes can be made without using *any* added oil. To avoid using oil, simply place a small amount of liquid in the bottom of the pan from the very beginning and cook, with the pan covered, over low heat.

Similarly, grain products contribute to weight gain and can be eliminated. Small amounts of grain products add flavor, but of the recipes standalone without the addition of extra carbohydrates.

All of the dishes can be modified to accommodate a gluten-free diet by using gluten-free grains or no added grains.

SOUPS AND CHOWDERS

In the popular child's tale, "Stone Soup," three hungry soldiers wander into a small town, commandeer a large pot, fill it with water, and place it in the center of town over a fire. Their only contribution to the pot is a stone. Attracted by the commotion, curious onlookers stroll by and ultimately add an ingredient. Before long, a rich hearty soup is bubbling away, enough to feed the entire community plus the three soldiers.

Soup is the ultimate one pot meal and is an excellent way to add nutritious foods to your diet. Homemade soups and stews are generally more tasty and substantial than those found in restaurants or out of a can, which are often mostly broth. Good for that day and the next, soup also freezes well.

Creating soup is simple. Place the ingredients into a large pot, cover with liquid, bring to a boil, and simmer for about 20-30 minutes. The list of ingredients can include almost any vegetables, meat, whole grains such as brown rice or barley, and herbs and other seasonings.

STANDARD AMERICAN FARE

Though fast-food and processed meals have changed everything, historically, a standard evening meal in America included a meat, a vegetable, and a starch. Meat often stood as the centerpiece. Having meat on the table symbolized affluence and was also considered healthful. Other food items were relegated to the edge of the plate. Envision a T-bone steak with a baked potato and separate bowl of iceberg lettuce salad covered in dressing. Times have changed. If, by this point, you still consider this to be a healthy meal, we still have some work to do.

These days meat needs to give up its place in the center and move to the sidelines. Meat can be a tasty addition to a meal, but just a small amount will do. Vegetables need a more prominent place; in fact, an assortment of several vegetables can make an adequate meal. Starch does not have to be completely eliminated, but it should have only a cameo appearance, never the starring role.

Envision a restaurant with a menu composed only of side dishes. For a meal, pick any two to three items from the list.

grilled wild salmon	steamed shrimp	chicken breasts
lean steak	baked sweet potatoes	baked red potatoes
tofu or tempeh	mashed cauliflower	rice and beets
rice and beans	slaw	

steamed vegetables *(any kind and any combination)*
baked beans *(homemade, not out of a can)*
scrambled eggs *with sautéed onions, peppers and tomatoes*
butternut/acorn squash
whole grains *such as barley or quinoa*
fresh potato salad with red potatoes
green peas with sautéed mushrooms
black eyed peas (without the fatback)
steamed or sautéed greens such as collards, kale or Swiss chard
sautéed mushrooms of different varieties

A meat with two or three different types of vegetables, such as butternut squash and steamed cabbage can make a perfectly acceptable meal. Eat fish and seafood more often. Plan some meals without using meat at all.

*For more suggestions and some additional recipe ideas, turn to the appendix section of this book. Recipes can also be found at **www.vitalplan.com**.*

COPING IN THE WORKPLACE

If your workplace is anything like the average, there is a constant stream of cakes, cookies, and pastries coming through the break area. The snack machines are full of honey buns, candy bars, soft drinks, and assorted other processed food items. They are hard to resist. Trying to avoid snacks completely is probably not a good idea, especially if weight loss is desired. Snacks provide an energy boost and a moment of relaxation, both of which are helpful in getting you through the day.

Going for snack foods that are healthful and nutritious generally means bringing your own. It also means getting used to snack foods that aren't traditional. See the previous section for some ideas. Make a habit of always bringing something to work or having something on hand. Your body will reward you for your discipline.

EATING OUT

Times are changing and fast-food restaurants are starting to add token "healthy" items to menu boards, but most offerings have low nutritional value. And eating a salad while everyone else around you is chowing down on cheeseburgers can be a real challenge. In most cases, typical fast-food restaurants are best avoided—though, admittedly, some are better than others. Many sit-down chain restaurants are stepping up to the plate with healthy offerings that are truly healthy, but more time is required for a meal.

For fast-food that is actually healthy, health food stores and grocery stores are the best bet. Many now have salad bars, delis, and quality food to go. Several chains of upscale groceries, such as Whole Foods, offer meal selections that rival anything made at home. Most cosmopolitan areas now have these types of groceries. In a pinch, a handful of fruit, or celery and carrots with hummus make an adequate meal or snack. When traveling, a small cooler kept in the back of the car allows full advantage of this resource.

In restaurants, be aware that most chefs rely on sugar and fat to make food appealing. This is true even in the best of restaurants. Expensive is not necessarily synonymous with healthy. Some of the healthiest meals out are often found in midrange restaurants, usually with an ethnic flair such as Thai, Indian, Japanese, or Mexican. Restaurants that make legitimate boasts of healthy menus are gradually becoming more common.

For a night out on the town, don't starve all day. Go ahead and eat a normal midday meal. That evening, consider ordering just a salad and an appetizer for your whole meal. Often these are the healthiest and lowest calorie items on the menu. The wine and the company can be just as good. Don't forget, you can always ask that an item be prepared in lighter fashion. Ask for double vegetables instead of rice or potatoes. I have never been turned down with this request. Maybe if enough people ask, restaurants will get the message. Consider sharing an entrée with another person or taking half home for another meal.

For something different, occasionally plan an extended lunch out with family or friends. Most restaurants serve lighter and healthier meals at lunch.

TRAVEL

Travel offers a wonderful opportunity to enjoy food. We traveled as much as possible when my kids were growing up. I always insisted that chain restaurants were to be avoided unless there were no other alternatives. This opened up a wide variety of fresh foods that were not available at home. Fresh salmon and blackberries in Oregon, cherries and apples in Washington State, artichokes and apricots in California, oranges and grapefruit in Florida, lobster in Maine. We sampled wherever we went. Local fare can, of course, be found at restaurants, but meals need not be confined to indoors, since items picked up at local markets and roadside stands can make great picnics along the way.

Food is often the centerpiece of experiencing new places and cultures. Add this pleasurable dimension to travel wherever you go.

SPECIAL OCCASIONS

The act of sharing a celebratory meal with friends and family can be a health experience in itself. Holiday meals can be made to be healthy. Just the fact that people tend to cook fresh food is a step in the right direction. Holidays tend to be centered on times when there are plenty of healthy foods available, such as citrus fruit, apples, pears, cranberries, and fresh nuts of many varieties. Try to keep the cookies and cakes to a minimum and be mindful of portion control and eating more slowly, but certainly do not let any of it get in the way of enjoying the food and the company. As long as celebratory feasting is reserved as a seasonal treat and not a weekly event, you should be able to indulge a bit!

Find more recipes in Appendix C, More Simple Cooking.

VITAL PLAN

Purify

Toxins are the most prevalent and insidious of all causes of disease. Removing toxins from the body is an essential step in achieving optimal health.

CHAPTER 10

Toxins, Microbes, and the Common Social Good

Carrot Island is a beautiful protected coastal area near my home. The marshes and bays are favorites for kayakers. Along with the beauty, there are mosquitoes. On any given day between May and December, there is a good chance of being bitten by one. A century ago the threat of malaria was very real. Because of the efforts of a Swiss chemist in the 1940's, I can regularly paddle these waters with no concern for contracting malaria. His discovery was a chemical pesticide that was inexpensive to produce, lethal to mosquito populations, easy to disseminate, and purportedly harmless to humans. Thousands upon thousands of lives were saved as malaria carrying mosquitoes were eradicated from much of the planet. In 1948, chemist Paul Müller was distinguished with a Nobel Prize for his discovery of the chemical pesticide DDT.

A scant fourteen years later, biologist Rachel Carson alerted the world to the adverse impact that DDT and other chemicals were having on the environment in her book, Silent Spring. As it turns out, DDT was not only lethal to mosquitoes but was lethal to all insects, even those vital to a balanced environment. It was later discovered that DDT also affected reproductive hormones in birds, such that the shells of their eggs were too thin and easily cracked, leading to an alarming plummet in certain bird populations. The potential for harm to humans was much greater than originally thought.

Rachel Carson spent her summers doing research on Carrot Island. At that time, the sight of a brown pelican was probably rare. Because of her efforts, my excursions around Carrot Island are complemented by flocks of brown pelicans skimming across the water and the sharp call of ospreys overhead.

THE COMMON SOCIAL GOOD

As a society we make decisions that affect our collective health and well-being. As individuals we can let our voices be heard to influence those decisions. Eliminating mosquitoes was a decision our society made to do away with a microbial threat; yet, in doing so, we created another threat. The DDT threat was resolved because of the alarm sounded by a single individual. Life is a give and take in which we each take a role. We all want the best in life and must work together to achieve that goal. This concept can be referred to as "the common social good."

The common social good has done much to change the standard of living in this country over the past hundred years. Epidemics of microbial infections, childhood illnesses, and secondary bacterial infections are much less of a threat than in the past. Modern antibiotics can be given some credit for this change, but the most influential factors have been improved standards of sanitation and the distribution of vaccines, both being decisions administered by our society as a whole. Seemingly simple concepts such as garbage collection, city sewers, and government bureaucracies that ensure that our cars, appliances, tools, etc. are safer are all aspects of the social infrastructure that have positive influence on our personal health.

Though the common social good has set a high standard of living in this country, all that we enjoy is still threatened. Some threats are invisible and hard to define. Who knows how much fallout from nuclear testing over the past 50 years has influenced our risk of cancer and chronic disease. And some threats seem to never completely go away: microbes will be around long after we are gone. One particular area where we could do a better job is reducing the hidden threat of toxins, but even that task is not straightforward.

The dichotomy of DDT as both friend and foe illustrates why eliminating certain threats to our well-being is so challenging. Toxic chemicals do not just appear. Their creation is associated with a purpose that generally enhances our lives in some way. Toxins may be intended products, as with chemical pesticides or cleaning agents, or they may be by-products, such as chemicals that leach into the environment with the manufacture and use of plastics or in vehicular exhaust.

A common link that many toxins share is an association with petroleum or other hydrocarbon fuel sources. Nonrenewable hydrocarbon energy sources, mainly consisting of petroleum and coal, are the ultimate source of the high living standards to which we have all become accustomed. Petroleum not only powers the planet but also provides for all of our needs and wants. Everything you see around you and everything you touch is associated with petroleum in some way. The carpet on the floor, the paint on the walls, the pen you write with, the dashboard in your car and the plastic bottle holding your beverage are all derived from petroleum. All of our food production is associated with petroleum-driven machines and petroleum-derived pesticides are used heavily in the industry. Even clothing involves petroleum: synthetics are oil-derived, and cotton is grown, harvested, spun, and sewn with the help of electricity that is at least partly oil based.

If petroleum were used more conservatively, it could be used to provide a high standard of living for hundreds of years into the future, without adversely affecting the environment. We would have to learn to live differently, but not necessarily less comfortably.

Because petroleum, natural gas, and coal provide for so much good in our lives, it is easy to overlook the fact that they are also the source of most toxins. As the rest of the world seeks the same standard of living that we enjoy in the industrialized world, the atmosphere is becoming increasingly saturated with toxins, and at the same time cancer and other chronic diseases of immune dysfunction are becoming alarmingly more common.

Just as a gas leak in a coal mine is not obvious to coal miners until it is too late, an increase in human disease from the insidious buildup of toxins in the environment can be difficult to recognize. Traditionally, coal miners used a canary to call alert to the possibility of impending disaster. In Rachel Carson's day, large birds were the "indicator species" for the adverse changes DDT was inducing in the environment. Today, two other groups of animals—amphibians and bees—may suggest that something equally sinister is happening in the earth's environment.

For many years scientists have been tracking a worldwide decline in all amphibian species (frogs and salamanders). This decline has not been limited to industrialized countries. It also has been occurring in amphibian populations deep in the rain forests of the world, suggesting that something is affecting our atmosphere. Though cause and effect has not been established, the decline parallels the increase in petroleum and coal usage worldwide.

Another alarming indicator of widespread environmental change is the worldwide decline in honeybee populations. Without these bees we lose the Garden of Eden: these proficient pollinators are a necessity for production of many of our fruits and vegetables. A recent Nature documentary on public television related the efforts of researchers to find the cause of the global decline in bees. Not surprisingly, they found not just one potential cause but multiple ones, culminating in a "perfect storm" of adverse conditions that may be contributing to a precipitous decline in hive populations. Pesticide use was very high on the list. Microbe infestation was common; this may be related to malnutrition and to the stress of being trucked frequently from farm to farm, following the needs of crop-growers.

Interestingly, as worldwide bee populations remain in decline, the hives of small organic beekeepers are stable and healthy. This observation suggests that if we are wise, we can have our cake and eat it too.

INDIVIDUALS CAN MAKE A DIFFERENCE

Walking or riding a bike is an obvious way to decrease pollution and is good for your personal health at the same time. Carpooling, driving a fuel-efficient car, or using mass transit make a positive statement. Conservation of electricity at home with thermostat adjustments and compact fluorescent bulbs is not only practical but also cost-effective.

Tax incentives make a solar hot water heater a better deal than ever before.

Being energy conscious and toxin aware does not necessarily mean giving up creature comforts. In 2005 my wife and I designed and had constructed a passive solar home. The overall cost was no more than any other conventional home of the same size. It is bright and warm, even on the coldest winter day. Our solar room is filled with plants most of the year. I even grow fresh herbs in the winter. The ventilation is such that only in the heat of middle summer do we turn on the air-conditioner. So far, our energy costs have been about half that of a conventional home of the same size. We made a decision to use non-toxic paints, even though they cost a bit more. We are careful about cleaners and pesticides. We installed a central vacuum to more effectively remove allergens. Such a home is truly a refuge from the outside world and a most pleasant place to live.

Another way to use less petroleum is by recycling. Recycling is not a new concept. Before 1950 and especially during World War II, everything that could be recycled was recycled. Liquids were contained in glass or tin and most other items were kept in paper or cardboard. Paper bags were the only option at the grocery store; most shoppers carried their own baskets. Milk was delivered to your doorstep in recycled glass bottles. Soft drinks, the newest drink craze, were available in recycled bottles.

In the 60's and 70's America was just learning to be a throw-away society. Paper trash and bottles littered our highways and byways. Many a young entrepreneur, including myself, earned pocket change by collecting discarded roadside bottles for the five-cent deposit. Those nickels added up. No matter where you happened to be, a ready supply of cash was always lying in the ditches, waiting to be harvested. Because of the simple five-cent incentive, a substantial percentage of those bottles ended up back at the bottler to be perpetually refilled. Though I seldom drink soft drinks any longer, I, for one, am sorry to see that bottle-deposits are no longer mandated in most states.

As our dependence on petroleum deepened, we became more and more of a throw-away society. Plastic containers of all varieties lie buried in our landfills and litter our public places. Unlike glass, which is inert, and paper, which is biodegradable, plastics will be shedding toxins to the environment for hundreds of years—not just on land but also in our oceans, lakes and rivers. Who knows what kind of toxic stew we are creating.

Part of the solution to the plastic problem is using less of it. Every time you wash your dishes instead of just throwing them away, you are recycling. Get back into the habit of drinking out of a glass instead of a plastic bottle. Store your water in glass whenever possible. When you need disposable cups, use paper ones (if you can find them) instead of plastic. At the grocery store, buy fresh food not wrapped in plastic whenever possible. Bring your own shopping bags. When you cannot reuse something yourself, recycle it through a waste management service. Recycling plastic not only conserves petroleum but also conserves energy.

Beyond decreasing our exposure to toxins, there are more pressing reasons to conserve petroleum. Our time in the Garden of Eden is running out. At present usage, petroleum flow will peak soon—perhaps this decade—and the remaining petroleum will be increasing difficult to extract. Natural gas will peak out at about the same time. Coal is much more plentiful, but is very dirty to use.

Many people seem confident that after petroleum and gas are gone, some other energy source will be "discovered," but make no mistake—there is no substitute. Petroleum is raw energy, made by ancient microbes and then encapsulated within the earth for millions of years. Alternative sources of energy, including wind, water, nuclear energy and biofuels, may help us prolong the blessing of petroleum but cannot replace it. Ironically, even alternatives depend on petroleum to some extent—for example, plastics are essential for construction of photovoltaic cells.

If petroleum sources were to suddenly dry up tomorrow, we would quickly plunge into the dark ages.

If we could learn to be better stewards of our Garden of Eden, it could be enjoyed by many generations to come. Simply by conservation, the blessings of petroleum could balance the problems associated with petroleum usage. For example, trains, instead of trucks, could be used to transport food and goods across the country with a fraction of the current energy expenditure. Using alternative sources of energy to reduce our dependence on oil and decreasing our total reliance on plastic would not only prolong the availability of our finite reserves of petroleum but would also slow global warming and significantly decrease the burden of toxins in the environment.

SELF PRESERVATION IN A WORLD OF HIDDEN THREATS

Certainly no one would ever think of intentionally drinking or eating pesticides, chemical cleaners, or industrial by-products, and yet we readily allow these substances to enter our homes, our food, and our water supplies. We are not aware because the quantities are too small to see or taste. Measured *independently,* small doses of chemical toxins may not produce immediate adverse effects, but *cumulatively* the story may be quite different.

The normal level of any toxin in the human body is <u>zero</u>!

Recent science studying concentrations of various toxins in human populations from around the country suggests that toxins do accumulate within the human body (http://pollutioninpeople.org). The human body seems to be a sponge for chemical toxins and tends to store many of them in our body fat. Common sense would suggest that chemical toxins do have potential for harm and probably do play a significant role in disease, but the question of "how much" is hard to answer because there are so many different toxins and the total load and interactions are hard to quantify.

Waiting around until someone defines the exact amounts of specific toxins the average person can tolerate is not practical, but becoming "toxin aware" is. Avoiding toxins in a toxin-filled world is not as difficult as it sounds. Toxic chemicals, allergens (substances that cause allergic reactions), and microbes can only enter the body in a limited number of ways. For instance, we can breathe them in, consume them via food and drink, or absorb them through our skin. Becoming aware of common sources of toxic substances and how they enter the body is the first step in decreasing their impact.

"GOOD" WATER

It is a sad fact that much of world's water supply is contaminated with chemical toxins, heavy metals, and microbes. In this country sanitation standards are currently high, but safe water is not guaranteed everywhere in the world. Water, however, is the easiest entity to fix. Any water can be filtered. Particulate and carbon filters (in-line or hooked up to the tap) remove the majority of contaminants, leaving water safe and drinkable.

Beyond filtration, the question of what constitutes healthy water is a matter of opinion. Minerals-out or minerals-in is central to the debate. All water from ground sources, either well or natural spring, contains dissolved minerals and is considered mineral water. Mineral content varies widely with geographic location. Traditionally, mineral water has been considered healthy, but health potential is highly dependent on the types of minerals dissolved in the water, as not all minerals are considered beneficial. There is also the matter of taste: certain minerals improve the taste of water and certain others do the opposite.

Calcium, the most abundant mineral found in groundwater, is considered desirable for healthy bones. Magnesium, common in water supplies but often deficient in food sources, is important for bone formation and normal cardiac function. Iron and copper, on the other hand, are probably best obtained from food sources, since the inorganic forms of iron and copper found in mineral water are not readily absorbed through the intestines. Sulfur compounds present in many groundwater sources give water an undesirable "rotten-egg" smell but are not necessarily harmful for consumption.

The presence of minerals defines water as being "hard." Removing minerals from water appears to be more about aesthetics than health. Since the 1930's, mineral residues (bathtub rings, etc.) have been considered unsightly and many households found in hard-water areas opt for a water softener. Water softeners use salts that substitute sodium for minerals found in the water. While soft water is less likely to leave stains on the tub and sink, the health benefits of softened water are questionable. Such water can add significant amounts of sodium to the diet.

In 2004, a World Health Organization expert consensus on water suggested that the healthiest water is hard water, filtered of any microbial and organic chemical contaminants, but still containing essential minerals, especially magnesium and calcium. Evidence cited in the consensus strongly suggests that incidences of heart attacks, cancer and other diseases are decreased with increased magnesium and calcium content in water supplies.

The composition of the water spilling from the tap in your home is highly dependent on the source. Well-water varies with location and depth of the well. Municipal water sources can be derived from wells drilled into underground aquifers or from surface waters, such as rain-fed reservoirs and rivers. Mineral content is highly variable and chemicals such as chlorine and fluoride are commonly added to municipal water. Some public water is highly suspect and some is quite good, with all gradations in between.

For your home, whether the water source is municipal or well, having the water checked for mineral content, pH and contaminants is a worthwhile endeavor. This can be done through any local health department. "Good water" would be defined as having moderate to high levels of calcium and especially magnesium with a slightly alkaline pH of 7.4. Excess iron and sulfur can be removed by special filtration systems. To decrease bathroom stains and scale, having a water-softener for the main house and a separate hard-water line for drinking water may be worthwhile. Drinking water can be filtered with simple carbon and particulate filters to remove any contaminants. Reverse-osmosis systems provide very safe water but also remove all minerals. The newest trend in R/O filtration, however, is a system that completely filters the water and then adds back the proper amounts of calcium and magnesium.

Another trend in water treatment is ionization. When mineral-containing water is exposed to an electrical current, the minerals within the water form negative ions and shift the pH toward alkaline. Alkaline mineral water is desirable, but before going out and spending a thousand dollars on one of these devices, have your water checked. If the magnesium and calcium levels are high and the pH is near 7.4, a water ionizer is not a necessity. If calcium and magnesium are not present or you have a water-softener, then the ionizer will not do you any good anyway. Note that distilled water or water run through a reverse-osmosis system has the minerals removed and will not ionize—unless the minerals are added back. If you want alkalized water and are averse to spending that amount of money, a poor-man's water ionizer is a teakettle. Water can be ionized by simply bringing it to a boil, as you would do for making tea.

Mineral water that has been alkalized by ionization or boiling is the tastiest water you can drink and possibly the healthiest. Alkalized water may be beneficial for decreasing the risk of osteoporosis, kidney stones and possibly gallstones.

If your best source of drinking water ends up being bottled water, take the time to research its origins (www.mineralwaters.org). The mineral content of commercially-sold bottled water is highly variable and dependent on where the water was acquired. Some bottled waters come from documented spring-fed sources, but many are simply municipal water that has been filtered, with minerals added. Though often criticized as not being "the real thing," the latter option may be the best because the water is highly filtered, with specific minerals added back in specific ratios. Groundwater may or may not contain the most desirable types and ratios of minerals, and, if not filtered, may contain contaminants.

Remember that chemicals from plastic bottles can gradually leach into the liquid stored in them. This is especially true if the container is heated. Whenever possible, store your water in a glass container. When plastic is the only option, keep your water bottle out of the sun and in a cool place. Aside from potential toxicity, the sheer load of plastic waste generated by this industry may be the biggest deterrent to bottled water. Hopefully the future will bring a return to recyclable glass containers for bottled retail beverages.

Beyond filtration, do your part to keep our water supplies clean and our landfills lighter. Using fewer disposable products and plastic products, eating organic and eating lower on the food chain translates into less pollution contaminating our streams, rivers, lakes and estuaries. Paper products are a significant source of water contamination. Toilet paper, napkins and paper towels are usually bleached with dioxins. Non-bleached and recycled paper products are becoming more widely available. The extra cost of these products is balanced by better health and a cleaner environment.

www.realgoods.com One of the oldest retailers of environmentally-sound products.

www.seventhgeneration.com Resource for safe cleaning products and non-bleached paper products.

When traveling to other countries, remember that water-borne microbial threats are common in many parts of the world. They are tied to different standards of sanitation and personal hygiene than we enjoy here. Local residents may have adapted to the microbes, but those germs are foreign to you. If you travel outside of this country consider purchasing a portable water filtration system. These can be found at any outdoor or camping supply store. You may look a little odd filtering your glass of water at the dinner table, but it may save you from a severe case of dysentery.

TOXIC CHEMICALS IN OUR FOOD

The steady rise in the types and concentrations of toxins in our food over the past fifty years is concerning. The primary culprits are large-scale commercial agriculture and commercial food processing. Industrial residues and by-products of plastics and petroleum also contribute to soil and water contamination. Fortunately, we are beginning to have some better choices. Organic produce and chemical-free products are becoming more readily available everywhere.

The overall cost of organic food is less than you would think. Though the retail cost of such food steers many away, it is a matter of supply and demand: As more individuals demand organic food, the cost will gradually come down—and our total healthcare bills will also likely substantially decrease. In addition, a switch to organic eating means that our water supplies and the environment in general would be safer and cleaner, an added benefit for every living thing on the planet.

The sheer numbers of potentially toxic molecules to which we are exposed on a daily basis is problematic. Even organically-produced food contains some natural toxins, and other toxins are difficult to eliminate from our soil and water. Many foods, even organically-produced ones, have the potential to cause food sensitivities. A wide variety of medical conditions can be caused or aggravated by sensitivities to certain foods. So, beyond organic, the keyword in healthy eating is diversity.

Eating a varied diet and rotating foods with the seasons is a naturally healthy practice. Make a habit of buying local produce whenever it is available. This helps small farms and decreases transportation costs and associated pollution. Get to know local farmers, many of whom are making efforts to decrease pesticide usage, even though they have not been officially "certified" as organic. It also makes sense to rotate food sources so as to reduce the cumulative impact of any one particular toxin that might be in a product.

One way to reduce your toxin load from food is to avoid products that are directly encased in plastic. Sometimes even organic foods come packaged in plastic. This may sound like paranoia, but the evidence linking chemicals leached from plastic to chronic disease and cancer is too great to ignore. Foods containing fats are especially vulnerable. Many chemicals associated with plastics and pesticides are hormonally active. Nicknamed "xeno-estrogens," these chemicals mimic estrogen in the body or affect the metabolism of estrogens, increasing the risk of hormonally-active cancers including breast, uterine and prostate cancer. Reducing exposure to xeno-estrogens is one of the primary ways to reduce the risk of cancer. Importantly, cruciferous vegetables, essential fatty acids, ground sesame seeds and ground flax seeds are several important foods for augmenting the ability of the liver to metabolize estrogens and xeno-estrogens in our "estrogen-dominated" environment.

Local markets and farmers markets where fresh vegetables and fruit are displayed in open bins are often the best places to buy your food. This may be your best opportunity to find the safest, freshest foods possible. When you go, bring your own cloth bags and a cooler for free-range meat. When shopping at a conventional supermarket, choose liquid food products in glass or paper containers whenever possible and avoid (to the extent practical) food products wrapped in plastic.

CHEMICALS FROM THE MEDICINE CABINET

People readily and voluntarily take pharmaceuticals every day but are unaware that most drugs could actually be classified as forms of toxins. Though they are sometimes lifesaving and useful in many ways, all drugs all have the potential for side effects and are metabolized within the body in the same way as any other toxins. In medical therapy we try to select beneficial effects of drugs over the toxic effects, but for most drugs eliminating the toxic effects altogether is impossible.

The fact is that the majority of synthetic drugs have been in use for less than fifty years—not even one human lifespan. Some of the more commonly used drugs have been approved for use within the past two decades, which is hardly enough time to determine the long-term potential for toxicity.

Gaining the most from pharmaceutical therapy while minimizing side effects is a matter of choosing the lowest dose possible and supporting therapy with appropriate lifestyle and dietary changes. Multiple drug therapy should be avoided whenever possible. Supplementation with high quality multivitamins is indicated because many drugs have the potential to induce vitamin and mineral deficiencies. Coenzyme Q-10, an important component in energy production, should be used in conjunction with any medications for cardiovascular or diabetic therapy.

Not infrequently I see patients with chronic disease who bring with them a long list of medications used to control their symptoms. In some cases I wonder whether their illness is more related to side effects of medications than to the actual disease process.

Though the vast majority of herbal therapies have been safely used by humans for thousands of years, there are a few exceptions. Commonly-used, over-the-counter remedies such as kava, hops, and valerian have been found to cause liver damage in certain individuals. St. John's wort, used for depression, can inhibit detoxification pathways in the liver and increase toxicity of other medications. Caffeine, found widely in nature, can cause insomnia and raise blood pressure in some people. It should be noted that many plants naturally contain toxic substances. Tobacco is a good example.

Seeking advice from someone knowledgeable about natural therapies increases therapeutic value and decreases the potential for toxicity.

Most people would not argue that illicit street drugs would fall in the category of being toxins. Many of them were originally used for medicinal purposes and some are available by prescription, but recreational use dictates higher (sometimes near-lethal) doses. The most commonly used recreational drug, voluntarily consumed by millions of people worldwide, is alcohol. Like most chemicals, toxicity of alcohol is determined by dose. At a lower dosage—say, a glass of red wine or a bottle of beer occasionally—alcohol actually has some health benefits, probably because of its mild anti-anxiety properties and the antioxidants in the wine or beer.

Another obvious source of self-inflected toxins is cigarette smoking. Approximately a third of Americans smoke, and a large proportion of them are young people. Many experts argue that smoking is our leading preventable cause of morbidity, but some evidence speaks to the contrary. In Europe, smoking is still popular and an interesting study documents that lean German vegetarians who smoke do not suffer morbidity significantly worse than non-smoking populations (Heidelburg Vegetarian Study). In this country, smokers tend to follow the worst health habits *and* the worst dietary practices—compounding all of their health concerns. Smoking *is* certainly bad for your health but possibly not as bad as the average American diet.

FOOD ALLERGIES

True food allergies are not as common as most people think. Food allergies can occur to any food and cause classic symptoms of itching, hives and, in severe cases, difficulty breathing. Top food allergies include: milk and milk products, eggs, peanuts, tree nuts, seafood, shellfish, soy, strawberries and wheat (gluten). Food allergies are generally easy to identify.

Sensitivities to foods occur more frequently. Most everyone can claim at least some sensitivity to some foods, with certain individuals plagued by multiple food sensitivities. Food sensitivities typically cause delayed symptoms of joint and muscle pain, fatigue and general achiness. Generally this situation results from a hyper-stimulated immune system associated with gastrointestinal dysfunction. Often this is precipitated by chronic and excessive consumption of wheat products, which damage the mucosal lining of the intestines. (More about this in the next chapter.)

MICROBES IN OUR FOOD

Microbes in our food can be either friend or foe. Our gastrointestinal tract depends on regular inoculations of favorable bacteria from fermented foods for normal function. Furthermore, without microbial fermentation we would not enjoy bread, yogurt, sauerkraut, blue cheese, wine, or beer.

Fermentation with the wrong microbes, however, can be quite threatening. A turkey sandwich left out on the counter overnight warrants a toss into the trash. Food spoilage may be obvious, which alerts a potential consumer, but the presence of undesirable microbes may also be subtle.

As mentioned earlier, many processed foods and certain uncooked foods are often colonized with unfavorable bacterial and fungal species that produce harmful toxins associated with an increased risk of cancer and immune suppression.

The food industry is generating a whole new set of concerns. Most livestock are fed unnatural foods and kept in confined quarters. This results in a high rate of disease that accounts for 70% antibiotics use in this country. Heavy antibiotic use selects for pathologic strains of antibiotic-resistant intestinal bacteria now being labeled as "super-bugs." Furthermore, the manure from the animals is sprayed on fields as fertilizer. Though it is only legal to spray before planting, some of these super-bugs are showing up in isolated outbreaks due to contamination of some crops.

HIDDEN TOXINS

There is mounting evidence that many types of pathologic microbes have the ability to take up residence in our tissues and remain hidden for long periods of time, sometimes for a lifetime. The mission of these microbes is simply to make more microbes: no intent to kill the host, only disable, allowing millions of microbial progeny to flourish. They do so by producing chemicals that compromise or control the host's immune and neurological systems. To us, these chemicals are toxins. Lyme disease may be the best known example of chronic disease caused by a hidden microbe, but there are many others. Research is suggesting microbial links to chronic diseases including as arthritis, chronic fatigue, sarcoidosis and possibly most of the autoimmune diseases.

We each harbor a perpetual struggle between the immune system and invading pathologic microbes whose sole purpose is commandeering our internal resources to ensure their survival. It seems we collect these microbes as we go through life; weighing us down and reducing our potential to recover from disease. Maintaining a healthy immune system by following good health habits is essential for staying ahead in the game.

Beyond good health practices alone, nature has provided additional protection in the form of herbal and other natural therapies. Many herbs and natural substances offer a broad range of antimicrobial properties. Garlic, andrographis, barberry, cat's claw and grapefruit seed extract are just a few examples. Modern science is now discovering ways to potentiate the value of these substances to protect us from a host of different types of microbial invaders. From everyday viruses that cause the common cold to superbugs created by antibiotic overuse, highly standardized and patented natural therapies are showing great value.

Heavy metals are another group of hidden toxins, with mercury being one of the most common. Mercury can be a factor in any chronic disease process, from hypothyroidism to heart attacks. The chief source of mercury in humans is amalgam dental fillings. Symptoms vary, but even if you just don't feel well, your amalgam fillings may be the problem. Replacing fillings can, however, be an ordeal; being checked for mercury toxicity first is a good idea. If mercury levels are high, dental fillings can be replaced. Replacement should be performed only by a qualified dentist specializing in extraction of amalgam fillings. After the source of mercury is removed, heavy metal detoxification should be carried out under the guidance of a qualified health practitioner.

The possibility of heavy metal toxicity should be considered if there is unexplained chronic disease. Furthermore, when chronic disease is present, toxins of any type (including heavy metals) are an impediment to healing. It is difficult to totally avoid exposure, but some individuals retain heavy metals to a higher degree than others. Body fat is the most important variable. Toxins of all varieties accumulate more readily in fatty tissue, another reason to stay as lean as possible.

Testing for toxin levels may be worthwhile in some cases, but defining toxicity is not straightforward (since the normal level of any toxin in the human body is zero). Reducing the level of toxins in the body is the best choice.

*The safest, most comfortable and possibly most effective way to remove common toxins, including heavy metals, from the human body is **far infrared (FIR) sauna**. Toxins are gently pushed to the surface and released through sweat. Often referred to as "healing waves," far infrared radiation is at the opposite end of the spectrum from damaging gamma rays and x-rays. FIR saunas are not exorbitantly expensive (about the price of a two-person hot tub) and can be installed in a home. The effectiveness and safety of FIR sauna is well documented in the scientific literature. FIR sauna is beneficial for many types of chronic disease and has been proven safe for cancer patients and patients with congestive heart failure.*

TOXINS IN THE AIR

Most of us spend much of our time inside tightly sealed air capsules. Our homes, workplaces, and automobiles are, for the most part, sealed from the outside environment. Whatever goes into these atmospheres stays and circulates. Toxic chemicals, microbes, and allergens can build up and become concentrated. The list includes numerous chemical toxins from plastics, paints, carpets and chlorinated cleaning products, and pesticides, dust, mites, molds, other microbes of many varieties, and many, many different types of allergens. The air inside an average home is often more toxic than the downtown air of a major city during summer.

AIRBORNE ALLERGENS

Many individuals are absolutely plagued by chronic sinusitis caused by allergies to dust, mold, and pollen of various sorts. When clinically tested, many of these individuals find that they are "allergic to everything." They spend their lives being chronically treated with antihistamines, nose-sprays, and rounds of antibiotics.

The underlying process is immune dysfunction, but the causes are the same as with any other disease—toxins, unhealthy food, microbes and chronic stress lead the list. And as with any other disease, treating the symptoms with drug therapy alone will not provide a cure. The real solution is restoring normal immune function. This is accomplished by decreasing or eliminating the causes—reduction of offending allergens is good place to start, but measures must also be taken to restore the balance of normal health.

The concept of an "allergy threshold" is very important. Most people do not become symptomatic until they reach a certain threshold of exposure. At this point, the immune system becomes overwhelmed and symptoms occur—a single trigger can be explosive. The most important way to avoid going over the threshold is by decreasing exposure. Allergy testing for not only airborne allergies, but also food sensitivities, can assist the individual in avoiding exposure to specific allergens.

The most obvious choice for reducing airborne allergens indoors is filtering the air. Air conditioner/heater filters should be changed every three months. Free-standing HEPA filter systems can be situated in rooms where most time is spent such as bedrooms and offices. Though outdoor air is not under personal control, knowledge of weather, ozone, pollen and pollution is readily available, and the choice can be made to stay inside!

Washing away allergens is another effective tactic. During pollen season, nasal washes with xylitol solution help to flush away allergens. Facial steam baths can help sooth mucous membranes in the nasal cavity. Try adding a drop or two of concentrated eucalyptus oil. Certain supplements taken on a regular basis during allergy season can optimize immune function and decrease the need for antihistamines and other pharmaceuticals. *Vitamin C, quercetin,* and *bromelain* are well known for calming the immune response to allergens. Probiotics (see next chapter) are important for restoring normal immune function.

Humidity that is too low or too high can adversely affect healing of sinus membranes. Ideal humidity is between 30 and 50%. Instruments to measure humidity are available at any hardware store. Properly functioning air conditioning lowers humidity and inexpensive room humidifiers increase humidity. Many people find that regular use of far-infrared sauna is very helpful in reducing symptoms.

Management of chronic allergies must extend beyond the nose. Symptoms associated with airborne allergies are frequently tied to gastrointestinal dysfunction and food sensitivities. Excessive consumption of wheat and dairy adversely affects intestinal function and contributes to hyper-stimulation of the immune system. Chronic emotional stress disrupts the balance of normal immune function and can be a major contributor to perpetuation of chronic allergies.

AIRBORNE MICROBIAL THREATS

A sneeze or a cough is all it takes to send a cold or flu virus toward its ultimate goal of infecting another victim. Contagious viruses and bacteria are spread by riding microscopic droplets of water carried through the air. The droplets can be inhaled directly or spread by contact after landing on countertops and food or sprayed into a telephone receiver. Constant vigilance by both the patient and others in the vicinity is required. Handwashing or use of an antimicrobial gel is essential, especially for those in the healthcare and food industries. Most important of all, however, is maintaining a healthy immune system.

Not to be overlooked, mold and mildew are invisible sources of misery for many people living in warm moist parts of the world. Mold spores are not only allergenic, but also have direct toxic effects. Toxic compounds, called mycotoxins, are secreted by certain mold species. Mycotoxins have to potential to not only irritate air passages and lungs, but also disrupt immune function causing a wide range of symptoms. Credited as the primary cause of "sick-building syndrome," mycotoxin-producing molds are significant hidden sources of ill health. Once the problem is identified, decontamination is best left to specialists, but in the short term, essential oils dispensed by a diffuser and HEPA filters can reduce the threat and improve living conditions.

TOXINS VIA THE SKIN

The outer layer of our skin, called the epithelium, provides a waxy coat that waterproofs and holds moisture in at the same time. Many substances, especially fat-soluble toxins, can be absorbed through the skin. Passage goes both ways, however, as sweating is one of the most effective ways to remove toxins and heavy metals from the body.

Modern humans spray on, rub on, and douse themselves in chemicals on a daily basis. The list of products that contain chemicals applied to the skin includes cosmetics, lotions, toothpaste, soap, shampoo, medicinal creams deodorants, and so on. Without a doubt, some of these chemicals have potential for toxicity, but as with chemicals allowed in our food, the level of toxicity is difficult to quantify. A partial list of commonly-used products recognized as having at least some potential for toxicity includes aluminum-containing antiperspirants, sodium laurel/laureth sulfate commonly found in soaps and shampoos, diethanolamine (DEA) found in many skin care products, propyl glycol found in many toiletry products, propyl alcohol used in mouthwash, toluene found in nail polish and perfume, and mineral oil made from petroleum.

Anything coming into contact with skin should be used with discretion. Some people are even sensitive to chemicals in toilet paper. Use skin care products judiciously and read labels. Natural is often better, but not always. Toxic chemicals occur in nature. Any products can contain substances that are allergens to certain individuals. Know your own body. Find products that work for you. The best way to keep your skin healthy is from the inside out. A healthy diet with balanced oils and sufficient antioxidants does more to keep skin healthy than anything else.

The final word on sunscreen is open for debate. The ionizing rays of the sun are a known contributor to skin aging and certain cancers[*], but many chemicals found in sunscreens can be classified as toxins. Sun exposure may

---

[*] Squamous and basal cell skin cancers have a definite link to sun exposure, but melanomas may not. As a gynecologist, having found melanomas between toes and other places where the sun doesn't shine, I tend to side with experts who suggest that melanomas may be more related to toxin exposure. Could it be that the rise in the incidence of melanomas is actually related to increased sunscreen use and not to increased exposure to the sun?

convert these substances into even more toxic compounds. As with many things, moderation and good judgment are essential. Carotenoids from regularly consumed vegetables protect from the inside out. Sleeves and a good hat may be your best sun protection.

When working with chemicals that are known toxins, such as paints, glues, or cleaners, always avoid direct exposure to the skin. Wear protective clothing and gloves. Do make sure that you have adequate ventilation.

I once burned my lungs while using bleach to clean mildew from the inside of an old sailboat. I had on protective gloves and clothing, but did not bother with adequate ventilation. It took several months before my lungs were completely back to normal.

EVERYDAY TOXIN AWARENESS

Exposure to toxins is continuous and cumulative. Toxin awareness is an important step toward decreasing the total toxin burden of the body. The following choices are easy and require minimal change in habits.

Tips for around the kitchen and bath

- Buy unbleached paper products—paper towels, napkins, tissues and toilet paper. Use washable cloth dish towels and cloth napkins whenever possible.

- Pots and pans: stainless steel is best. Aluminum and non-stick should be avoided. Cooking and drinking directly from copper or brass should be avoided.

  Iron and copper from organic sources (i.e., food) are essential for life, but free iron and copper ions in the bloodstream convert oxygen free-radicals into "super" free-radicals—a significant risk factor for atherosclerosis.

- Never microwave foods contained in plastic or wrapped in plastic wrap—especially fatty foods! Heated plastics out-gas chemicals which are readily absorbed into fatty foods. Microwave foods in glass or ceramic containers. Do not marinate foods in plastic bags.

- Plastic storage containers for foods are a necessity, it seems, but should be mostly limited to the refrigerator or freezer.

- Disposable plates and cups should be paper instead of plastic or Styrofoam.

- Nontoxic natural cleaning agents are widely available. Look for them at health food stores. Avoid cleaners containing chlorine and chlorinated compounds. Many natural and inexpensive cleaning options are available for around the kitchen and bath. Baking soda (mild abrasive), white vinegar, rubbing alcohol, ammonia, lemon juice, grapefruit seed oil, soap flakes and water are some examples. A simple, non-toxic household cleaner can be made from a half cup of ammonia solution, one pint of isopropyl alcohol, and a few drops of dishwashing liquid mixed in a gallon of water. White vinegar is excellent for cleaning windows.

  Other natural cleaners and non-toxic solutions can be found in the Reader's Digest book, *Homemade—How to Make Hundreds of Everyday Products You Would Otherwise Buy.*

- Scrutinize all toiletry products for potential toxicity. Avoid antiperspirants with aluminum if possible.

TIPS AT HOME

- Avoid using carpet in your home, especially if you have chronic allergies. If you buy carpet, opt for less toxic varieties with less "out-gassing" of chemicals. Most manufacturers provide specifications. All you have to do is ask. Carpets made from natural materials are available, but still readily collect hair, dust and dirt. Cork flooring does not collect dirt and is warm and soft on the feet; it may be the least toxic alternative.

- Nontoxic paints, wall, and floor coverings are more expensive, but are worth the cost.

- Choose minimally toxic ways to deal with pests and bugs. **Never allow someone to spray pesticides inside your home or office. These chemicals are extremely threatening and stay around for a long time.**

Use baits instead of widespread chemicals for eradicating pests. They are just as effective.

- Dust mites can be minimized with regular damp dusting. Many microscopic insect pests live in bedding. Wash linens and clean upholstery regularly. Consider placing a free-standing HEPA air filter in the room where you sleep, to avoid deep-breathing dust and other allergens all night.

- Change A/C filters frequently. Consider installing a whole house air filtering system. High-quality individual room filters can also be purchased. Look for filtering systems containing charcoal, particulate and HEPA filters. These are readily available for reasonable prices at home supply stores.

- Periodically have the duct work in your house completely cleaned by a professional.

- Negative ion generators. Negative ions inhibit free radicals derived from the harmful aspects of oxygen and air-borne pollutants. Negative ions exist naturally in air found over and around bodies of water. Possibly this is why a vacation at the beach or beside a lake feels soothing and healthy. Negative ion generators do have the ability to clean the air, but not as thoroughly as a HEPA filtering system; in some incidences, both are necessary. Negative ion generators can be found on the Internet and most home supply stores. When purchasing a negative ion generator, make sure it is "ozone-free."

- Central vacuum cleaners do the best job of actually removing dirt and dust completely from the house, but some better quality free-standing vacuums can also do the job.

- One-third of Americans still using tobacco products for relaxation and recreation. Smoking inside an enclosed air space affects everyone in that space. Cigarette smoke is a primary source of the toxic heavy metal cadmium. Because of pesticide use, tobacco products are probably more toxic than they were a hundred years ago.

   If you are a smoker, the need to quit goes unsaid; yet, before you do, there is one often unrecognized benefit of smoking that must be addressed. Smoking releases stress. Deep breathing and concentrated focus associated with smoking is extremely relaxing. Many people depend on smoking for stress management. When stopping smoking, other methods of stress reduction must be cultivated. Medications can be helpful but have significant side effects. Hypnosis and exercise are very beneficial for most people who are trying to quit.

COPING IN THE WORKPLACE (AVOIDING "SICK BUILDING SYNDROME")

- Office buildings often have poorer air quality than homes. In the South, mold in buildings is almost a given. Mold and mildew are especially common in large buildings. Most air filtering systems in large buildings are not satisfactory. Consider purchasing a high quality room air filter and possibly a negative ion generator to protect your own workspace.

  New buildings are not immune to the mold problem. I know of an office that was of new construction and yet, after only one year, the ceiling tiles were removed to reveal that all of the spaces above were saturated with mold.

- If you work in an industrial setting, be proactive about ensuring that ventilation systems and protective clothing meet the mark. Do not assume that you are protected. Voice your concerns tactfully but vigilantly. Remember that the management is interested in the bottom line and any regulations they have to comply with—not your health.

EXERCISES IN "TOXIN AWARENESS"

- Have your water tested. Install some type of water filter for drinking water.

- Spend a Saturday morning going through cabinets and under counters, reading labels of products in your home. Chlorinated products, products with threatening chemical ingredients, or products that just smell toxic should be noted. With a piece of tape and a pen identify these products as toxic. As they are used up, try to replace them with less toxic alternatives.

- On another Saturday evaluate personal products for potential toxic substances, such as aluminum in your deodorant. Try some of the natural brands of toiletry products to see if they work as well for you.

- Set up a calendar to change the filters in your air vents regularly. The same may apply to water filters and free-standing air filters. Remember to write the date on the filter itself.

- Consider purchasing a free-standing air filtering system for your office or workspace.

- Make a list of ways you could use alternatives to plastics in your everyday life and try to stick to it. Plastic has moved into a position of being nearly essential in our modern world, but recognize that all plastic has a least some potential for toxicity.

RADIATION AWARENESS

Radiation is the most invisible threat of all. Background ionizing radiation from the sun, the universe and the earth itself has been a present, but stable, force of disease since life began on earth. How much this threat has been accentuated by atomic bomb testing within in past 70 years and exposure to x-ray devices is completely unknown. Fortunately, the damage caused by ionizing radiation is very similar to oxidative stress, and protection can be gained from antioxidants found in foods and natural herbal therapies—just another reason to eat your vegetables and take your supplements every day!

Non-ionizing or electromagnetic (EM) radiation does not directly inflict measurable damage to tissues, but may be a significant threat, just the same. Like a science fiction movie come to life, we are surrounded by machines 24/7 and continually bathed in sea of electromagnetic radiation. Even our indoor recreational places are crowded with exercise machines churning out EM radiation. Logic would suggest that conflicting energies could disrupt the energy fields composing and surrounding the human body—how much, again, is a matter for debate. The best solution to the problem is intermittent avoidance. Periodic infusions of fresh air and open space are good for anyone and everyone!

Possibly the most prevalent concern for radiation exposure is a cell phone pressed to the side the head. Cellular phones emit electromagnetic radiation in the microwave range. Regular use of cell phones has been inconclusively linked to cancer, primarily brain tumors. While this risk has not been well defined and no one is suggesting given up cell phones, there are some simple precautions for decreasing exposure.

- Use remote wireless headsets and car speaker/microphone kits whenever possible.
- Text instead of talk (except while driving, of course)
- Do not charge a cell phone directly beside the bed.
- Do not carry a cell phone in a pocket with close contact to skin

Exposure to toxins, microbes, radiation, and other environmental stresses is nearly unavoidable. By making choices and changing our lifestyle, we can decrease our exposure, but the issue goes beyond avoidance strategies alone. Maintaining the body's internal waste removal and detoxification systems is essential for good health. The next chapter will address this important topic.

CHAPTER 11

Detoxification and Elimination

Silent, but deadly, toxins are significant contributors to disease. Toxins increase oxidative stress and disable the immune system, allowing microbes to set up shop. Toxins poison biochemical reactions, disturbing essential functions in the body. Though completely avoiding toxins is nearly impossible, we can choose to reduce our exposure. We can also support our bodies' intrinsic strategies for detoxification and elimination, without which toxins accumulate within our tissues.

Most toxic substances are fat soluble and are retained in fatty tissues. We depend mainly on the liver to convert these fat-soluble substances into less toxic water-soluble substances that can be removed more easily. This is a hard job. As we age, the liver becomes less efficient at detoxification and other functions such as regulating cholesterol and glucose. Liver cells that have sustained significant damage are gradually replaced with fat. Insulin-resistance from excessive consumption of carbohydrates (chiefly wheat and corn) compounds the problem by accelerating accumulation of fat in the liver. A taxed liver will develop a yellow color and is referred to as a "fatty liver."

Protecting liver function as we age is extremely important. The detoxification process produces significant oxidative stress and regular intake of antioxidants helps protect liver cells. Regular consumption of cruciferous vegetables (e.g., broccoli, cabbage, Brussels sprouts, kale, bok choy, and cauliflower) aids in removal of hormones and hormone-like toxins from the body, a significant factor in decreasing the risk of hormonally-active cancers such as breast and prostate. *Milk thistle* and *dandelion* are herbs well known for protecting liver function. Supplements containing these ingredients should be considered by anyone with a history of liver damage, individuals who are on numerous medications, and possibly anyone over the age of fifty.

After processing by the liver, by-products of the detoxification process must be removed from the body. There are three main pathways for removal: the colon, kidneys, and sweat glands. (A minor mechanism is exhalation.) Different toxins are processed in different ways. The majority of toxins are removed through the colon but others specifically exit via the urine. Some toxins can be removed directly by sweating, even before they pass through the liver. Working up a good sweat by exercising regularly or by using a sauna is a natural and important way to remove toxins.

The necessity of regular sweating has been recognized for ages. For populations around the equatorial regions, sweating throughout the hot day was a normal part of life, but for people in colder regions this was less true. Sweating had to be initiated. Native North Americans regularly participated in rituals that involved sweat houses. Saunas have been popular in Finland since the Middle Ages. Their use has now spread worldwide.

The vast majority of toxins are removed through the gastrointestinal system. After being processed by the liver, partially detoxified substances are carried by bile into the intestines and colon. Bile, consisting mainly of bile salts made from cholesterol, is secreted by the liver to help break down fat. Bile is tightly recycled in the body: 95% of bile is reabsorbed from the small intestine. *Most toxins can also be reabsorbed. This is where dietary fiber is so important.* Dietary fiber, made of indigestible material in our food, surrounds toxins that are in the intestine, thus preventing their reabsorption. How much fiber is necessary? The bulk of our food should be made up of fiber, but for average American, this is rarely the case: most Americans consume only about 5 to 10 grams of fiber daily, only a fraction of the 25 to 35 grams felt to be necessary for optimal health.

There are two types of fiber—soluble and insoluble. Soluble fiber holds water-soluble toxins within the colon for removal. Insoluble fiber makes up the bulk of feces; this type of fiber helps to push everything through. Fiber from vegetable sources is the best, overall. Dietary fiber also provides for removal of excess cholesterol from the system. (Inhibited flow of bile may be a contributing factor to rising blood cholesterol as we age.) Both types of fiber are important for normal gastrointestinal function and toxin elimination. Drink plenty of water as you increase your fiber intake.

Gastrointestinal function in general is intimately tied to our overall health. Our neurological system is tightly intertwined with our gastrointestinal system and much of our immune system resides within the gastrointestinal system. Not only is the gastrointestinal system responsible for digestion of food and removal of toxins, it encounters microbial invaders and potential allergens on a continual basis. *When the gastrointestinal system is out of balance or not functioning properly, every system in the body is affected.* The biggest enemies of normal gastrointestinal function are processed foods (with high sugar, starch, and fat content, but low dietary fiber) and emotional stress. These seem to go together all too often.

Emotional stress shifts the resources of the body toward dealing with the stress at hand and away from dealing with everyday matters such as digestion. Chronic emotional stress almost always results in gastrointestinal dysfunction. Poor nutrition adversely affects both the integrity of the lining of the GI tract (called the mucosa) and our ability to produce the enzymes necessary to break down food. Lack of fiber slows motility (the movement of food through the GI tract) even further and allows the buildup of toxins and abnormal bacteria in the intestines.

When our primitive man was escaping from a tiger, digesting food was the least of his body's concerns. Resources were temporarily shifted away from the gastrointestinal tract and toward the brain and muscles. If he happened to stop by a drive-thru during the escape, the burger would sit undigested in his stomach and begin to ferment. Gas produced by fermentation would be forced into the esophagus, carrying stomach acid along with it. Proper digestion would not resume until the stress eased off.

Most Americans live this way on a daily basis. They come home from a day of "escaping the tiger" to immediately sit down to the largest meal of the day—at a time when the GI tract is least prepared to deal with it. Consuming food when gastrointestinal function is suppressed leads to disastrous consequences.

STOMACH

For many people the stomach is where all health problems begin. Gastro-esophageal reflux and gastric ulcers are some of the most commonly treated disorders today. Chronic gastric dysfunction leads to erosion of the lining (mucosa) of the stomach, allowing ulcers to develop. The damaged tissues become fertile ground for secondary bacterial infections, most commonly *Heliobacter pylori*.

What happens in the stomach can greatly affect the other organs, including the esophagus. Poor eating habits, processed food, and stress delay gastric emptying, allowing food to stagnate and ferment. Gas and belching splash acidic liquid into the esophagus, causing inflammation and irritation of the esophagus. Painful erosions at the lower esophagus are part of *gastro-esophageal reflux disease (GERD)*.

Most treatment protocols assume that increased stomach acid is the total cause of the problem and focus therapy on suppressing it completely. In actuality, stomach acid is an essential ingredient of normal digestion and without it, digestion of food is compromised. Without stomach acid, proteins are not properly broken down for digestion. Important minerals and some vitamins are not properly absorbed. Threatening microbes pass through this normally impenetrable barrier unharmed. Food stagnates in the stomach and gastric motility is slowed. This, by itself, contributes to further mucosal damage. Minimally-digested food is eventually allowed to pass into the small intestine, causing problems further down the line.

Interestingly, as the incidence of gastric reflux has gone up in America, the incidence of stomach cancer has actually gone down. What was a common cancer a hundred years ago is now relatively uncommon. The reason has to do with a shift in food preservation. Prior to refrigeration, many foods, especially meats, were salted. Heavily salted foods are very rough on the stomach mucosa. Mainland Japanese still have a strong taste for salt and correspondingly have a relatively high rate of stomach cancer.

Erosions within the stomach are called *gastric or peptic ulcers* and present with classic "heartburn" symptoms along the left side of the upper abdomen. Erosions of the duodenum, where the stomach empties into the small bowel, are termed *duodenal ulcers*. "Infections" with the bacterium, H. Pylori, are often associated with peptic ulcers. These ulcers present with pain in the middle of the abdomen in an area called the "epigastric region" and can radiate to the back. All of these ulcers have the same origins and respond to the same therapy.

The first step in maintaining a healthy stomach is following a diet made up of a wide diversity of fresh vegetables and other natural whole foods with sufficient fiber. Regular consumption of fermented foods such as yogurt is an important practice for replenishing the normal bacteria of the entire gastrointestinal system. If esophageal or gastric irritation is present, acidic foods such as citrus and tomatoes should be avoided. Spicy foods such as hot peppers can irritate an established problem, but are not causative. Salt should be avoided. Coffee is a gastric irritant and tea is a mild gastric irritant. Caffeine increases production of stomach acid. Alcohol consumption aggravates established gastric disease.

The American habit of sitting down to a large meal at the end of a stress-filled day encourages gastrointestinal dysfunction. We would all do well to mimic our European neighbors with a main midday meal and a light supper, but most Americans find it hard to make the change. At the very least, a regular practice of distributing food throughout the day instead of a large end-of-day meal is better for digestion. Relaxing and stretching before a meal is another good practice.

When you sit down to eat with a group of people, are you the first to finish or the last? If your answer is first, insufficient chewing is likely a large part of any gastrointestinal upset you may be experiencing. Remembering that digestion starts in your mouth; make a conscious effort to eat more slowly and chew your food thoroughly. Chewing is the only part of the digestive process over which we have voluntary control. Completely chewing food may have more bearing on the incidence of digestive problems than anything else. Overeating is also less common in individuals who eat slowly and chew their food adequately, and it makes for a relaxed meal, which is better for digestion all the way around. A relaxed lifestyle in general has a positively influence on gastrointestinal function.

Large amounts of cold liquids consumed with food slow enzymatic function and impede digestion. Small sips of liquid during a meal are preferred. Again the Europeans are one up on us with a habit of drinking water, wine or beer at room temperature. Large iced drinks should be reserved for quenching thirst after exercise. This advice sounds harsh for most Americans, but it will reduce gastrointestinal dysfunction.

Dietary supplements should be considered before resorting to drug therapy. Since activation of digestive enzymes is compromised by a dysfunctional stomach, supplements containing enzymes to break down starches, sugars, proteins, and fat carry little potential for harm and may offer significant benefit. If bloating and stomach gas are prevalent, then reduced acid may be the problem. Try taking a couple of tablespoons of apple-cider vinegar in water with the meal—this strategy has helped many people with reflux.

Favorable bacteria, whether acquired from food sources or probiotic supplements, suppress the growth of secondary infections with harmful bacteria and fungal species. Bismuth subsalicylate, the ingredient found in the well-known over-the-counter remedy Pepto-Bismol, coats the mucosa and offers anti-inflammatory benefits; it effectively reduces secondary infections by the bacterium H. pylori. Deglycyrrhizinated licorice (DGL) and slippery elm are natural substances that can protect the mucosal lining. Antacids containing calcium and magnesium help, too.

SMALL INTESTINE

After being exposed to the acidic environment of the stomach, food enters the small intestine where the acid is neutralized. Partially digested food is now exposed to more digestive enzymes and to bile, secreted by the liver. Partially digested proteins, carbohydrates and fat are further broken down into component parts for absorption through the mucosa of the small intestine. If the digestive processes of the stomach or small intestine are compromised, partially-digested food is at risk of becoming putrefied by bacterial fermentation, rather than being properly digested—with gas and distension as the immediate result. Consumption of processed food, lacking natural enzymes that aid digestion, compromises the digestive process even further. Undigested and contaminated food materials activate the immune system and cause further problems.

Enzymes are key to the digestive process. Specific enzymes are secreted in order to break down most carbohydrates (except fiber), fats and proteins. As we age, digestion of proteins is compromised by reduced gastric acid secretion and gradual decline of digestive enzyme secretion. Digestion suffers and the incidence of gastrointestinal disorders increases.

Digestive enzymes are also naturally found within raw fruits, raw vegetables and raw meat. Pineapple and papaya are well known for containing digestive enzymes. These additional enzymes provide, for us, a boost to the digestive process. Processed and overly cooked foods contain no natural enzymes; this is likely another factor that contributes to the high incidence of gastrointestinal disorders seen today.

The enzymes naturally found in foods may have purpose beyond digestion alone. In Japan, a fermented soy product called "natto" is widely consumed. The bacteria in natto produce an enzyme, now called "nattokinase." When consumed by humans there is good evidence that nattokinase actively dissolves fibrin, the fibrous part of an arterial plaque—possibly one reason the Japanese are known for having the lowest rates of stroke and heart disease in the world. Other enzymes found in foods are known to have anti-inflammatory and analgesic properties in human consumers.

Under normal circumstances, foreign molecules such as proteins occasionally pass through the digestive process intact. Undigested proteins could represent a potential microbial threat or a potential allergen. Allowing such substances to cross the intestinal barrier into the bloodstream is very undesirable; thus, the immune system acts as a line of defense, ready and able to neutralize any foreign substance—especially foreign proteins. Because these food-based threats are relatively common, much of the immune system (70%) resides within the gastrointestinal system.

When digestion is compromised, undigested proteins pass in mass into the small intestine. Exposure to this flood of foreign proteins quickly overwhelms the local intestinal immune system. A call for help goes out from immune cells localized in the intestines to the immune system at large. Defensive cells congregate in the wall of the intestine to neutralize the threat. Resulting inflammation damages the intestinal mucosa, thus allowing foreign proteins to pass into the blood stream. Commonly referred to as *"leaky gut syndrome,"* the resulting inflammation is a contributing factor to *inflammatory bowel disease.*

Chronic consumption of modern wheat products seems to be an inciting factor in many incidences of leaky gut. Other food sensitivities may be associated when the process becomes established, but leaky gut is unusual in individuals who do not consume any wheat products. Whenever leaky gut is suspected, wheat products (refined white flour, whole grain wheat, and other gluten-grain products) should be strictly avoided to allow the gut to heal.

Proteins crossing into the bloodstream that have been neutralized by the immune system form "inflammatory complexes." These complexes are circulated throughout the body, causing symptoms well outside of the gastrointestinal tract. Unusual symptoms, such as fatigue, body aches, chronic skin conditions, headaches, muscle pain, joint pain, and even insomnia may result. Though wheat is a common instigating factor, once the process of leaky gut is established, sensitivities can occur to proteins of commonly consumed foods. This is the basis of food sensitivities. Sensitivities are often challenging to define because onset of symptoms is typically delayed for one or two days after the time an offending food is consumed. Fortunately, once steps are taken to heal the gut, sensitivities gradually resolve.

Food sensitivities associated with leaky gut syndrome should be differentiated from classic food allergies. True food allergies are associated with acute symptoms of itchy skin, swelling and watery eyes, and are relatively uncommon. The offending foods are normally easy to recognize and can be avoided. Generally a person will have allergies to one or only a few different types of foods. True food allergies are associated with a different type of immune reaction, last for a lifetime and are not necessarily associated with gastrointestinal dysfunction.

Bowel dysfunction with associated food sensitivities increases the body's total immune burden. Unrecognized food sensitivities, when combined with airborne allergies, push the immune system toward the breaking point referred to as the "allergy threshold." For this reason, nasal allergies and chronic sinusitis are commonly found in association with gastrointestinal dysfunction and food sensitivities.

Food sensitivities can produce symptoms beyond gastrointestinal dysfunction. Vegetables in the "nightshade" family including tomatoes, eggplant, potatoes, and peppers are notorious for aggravating arthritis. Some foods have a reputation for triggering migraines. Classic examples include caffeine-containing foods, red wine with sulfites, preserved meats containing sodium nitrite, dairy, chocolate, and foods containing the flavor-enhancer MSG. Problem foods and types of reactions can vary widely from person to person.

The first step in management of food sensitivities is recognition. Blood tests for acute food allergies and delayed-reaction food sensitivities can sometimes be helpful, but an elimination diet is often the best way to recognize and avoid offending foods. Gluten (wheat and related grains) and milk proteins are the most common offenders. Tree nuts and peanuts cause reactions in many people. With time, after the bowel has an opportunity to heal and the immune system is calmed, some foods can carefully be reintroduced on a limited basis.

LIVER, GALLBLADDER, AND PANCREAS

These three organs are intimately tied to each other and to the elimination process. Ducts from the liver, gallbladder and pancreas join to form the common duct which connects to the upper part of the small intestine. The liver secretes bile, which is necessary for the breakdown of fat. An extra supply of bile is stored in the gallbladder for use when excess dietary fat is consumed, such as after eating a double chili cheeseburger. The pancreas secretes enzymes necessary for digestion of everything else.

The flow of bile is a key point in the detoxification cycle. Once the liver cells have extracted fat-soluble toxins from the bloodstream and converted them into less toxic substances, they are shuttled into the bile. The rate of toxin removal is therefore dependent on the flow of bile. Stress and the consumption of processed foods, which tend to be inflammatory, inhibit the flow of bile.

Bile is made up predominantly of bile salts derived from cholesterol. Besides carrying toxins from the liver, bile is necessary for digestion of fat. Bile is dumped into the intestine, but then reabsorbed (recycled) later down the line. At that point, any water-soluble toxins that are not surrounded by indigestible fiber are also reabsorbed; thus, high-fiber diets expedite toxin removal from the body.

The brown color of stool represents bile. Light-colored stools suggest sluggish bile flow or excessive reabsorption of bile. Constipation, as you can surmise, is a risk factor for toxin retention. Loose stools, however, do not necessarily represent adequate flushing of the liver. Often bile flow is inhibited in disorders such as irritable bowel syndrome, and undigested fat contributes to diarrhea. "Congestion of the liver," with decreased bile flow, is very likely is a factor in many chronic disease processes, from elevated cholesterol associated with atherosclerosis to cancer.

The most common threat to this three organ complex is gallbladder disease. Extra bile is stored in the gallbladder. Gallstones, consisting predominantly of bile salts, form when the flow of bile is stagnant. Hereditary factors increase the risk of stone formation, but the most significant contributing factors are poor dietary habits and poor health habits in general. The stones themselves are generally not a problem, unless they become lodged in the common duct, completely blocking the flow of bile from the liver and causing painful back-up of enzymes from the pancreas.

LOWER SMALL INTESTINE AND COLON

Finally we get to the lower portion of the GI tract where the final processes of digestion, toxin removal, and elimination of waste material occur. The concentration of bacteria in this region is truly astounding and easily exceeds a trillion bacterial cells in adults with normal GI activity. Over 1000 different species of bacteria have been defined as normal flora in the gastro-intestinal system. An individual may harbor up to 150 of those species, but the assortment within one individual's bacterial flora may be quite different than that of another person.

The bacterial makeup of a person's gastrointestinal bacterial flora is almost as individual as his or her genetic code.

The bacteria of the colon (the first part of the large intestine) feed upon any undigested food particles remaining at this point and assist in the further breakdown of any toxins present. Gastrointestinal bacteria are also important because they produce certain vitamins essential for human health. When out of balance, overgrowths of abnormal or harmful bacteria can produce excessive gas and toxins, which cause pain and can actually slow or stop the elimination process— thus producing the miserable state of constipation.

Poorly digested food, low quality food, and slow motility promote overgrowths of abnormal bacteria in the colon, a condition that is commonly referred to as "dysbiosis." This process is further aggravated by a low-fiber diet, which lacks the bulk necessary to push toxic buildup of bacteria on through.

Slow intestinal motility often allows abnormal bacteria to backup into the small intestine causing gas and damage to the mucosa of the lower small intestine. I have commonly witnessed this phenomenon in patients who present with pain in the right lower portion of the abdomen, where the small bowel inserts into the large bowel. These patients are sometimes seen in the emergency room with symptoms similar to appendicitis. Most often this problem waxes and wanes through a person's lifetime and is a hallmark sign of irritable bowel syndrome.

"Dysbiosis" and "leaky bowel syndrome" are the roots of irritable bowel syndrome, inflammatory bowel disease and chronic constipation. When the digestive process is compromised upstream, problems in the large colon are often going to follow. Poorly digested processed foods feed abnormal bacteria. Overgrowths of abnormal bacteria produce gas and toxins that slow intestinal motility. Distension and discomfort result. The initial result is often constipation, but, as toxins build up, episodes of explosive diarrhea occur. The condition is referred to as *irritable bowel syndrome* (IBS). Some suffers have more of a tendency towards constipation and others toward frequent loose stools. Fortunately, however, damage to the mucosa is not usually severe and inspection of the bowel by colonoscopy typically reveals normal tissues.

Inflammatory bowel disease occurs when severe inflammation and ulceration of the mucosa are present. Inflammation and ulceration occurring randomly along the intestinal/colon tract is typically found in *Crohn's disease.* When the colon is affected primarily, the condition is called *ulcerative colitis.* Ulcerative colitis is more apt to be associated with a pathologic strain of bacteria that has taken hold in the colon.

Toxins produced by overgrowths of unfavorable bacteria can have far-reaching effects. Symptoms commonly associated with chronic fatigue and fibromyalgia may be related to dysbiosis. Breast cancer and arthritis may have links to dysbiosis.

Chronic constipation can include irritable bowel symptoms or exist by itself. Constipation occurs when the muscular contractions that move material through the colon are slowed or stopped. This process of intestinal motility, referred to as peristalsis, can be compromised by many things, including toxins in the food we eat, toxins produced by abnormal bacteria in the colon, and chronic distension of colon. Many medications also slow intestinal motility.

The good news is that there are many ways to reduce the severity of most GI disorders. Following a diet made up of a wide diversity of whole foods with sufficient vegetable-source fiber is important for maintaining a healthy lower gastrointestinal tract. Regular consumption of fermented foods such as yogurt replenishes favorable intestinal bacteria. Management of stress and regular practice of relaxation techniques are also essential for allowing the gastrointestinal tract to perform its job.

Restoration of normal gastrointestinal function is essential for overcoming any type of chronic health problem. Strategies for overcoming intestinal dysfunction should include recognizing and eliminating foods causing food sensitivities, aiding digestion with digestive enzyme supplements, soothing and protecting the intestinal mucosa with selected supplements, increasing dietary fiber to push abnormal bacteria through the tract, and replacing bad bacteria with favorable (normal) bacteria.

Supplements that may be beneficial include slippery elm, aloe vera juice and ginger tea (all soothe the intestinal mucosa), digestive enzymes, probiotic supplements and fiber supplements. The type of fiber consumed does matter. Vegetable fiber from natural food is preferred. Fiber from grains including oats, barley, brown rice and buckwheat is generally well tolerated. Wheat fiber, especially whole grain wheat fiber, is not tolerated well by many individuals and often causes gas. Fiber found in onions, leeks, garlic Jerusalem artichoke and asparagus feed favorable bacteria in the colon. This special type of fiber has earned the term "pre-biotic" and is found in supplement form.

Though psyllium is a natural grain product that is found in many natural fiber laxative supplements used for constipation, it causes gas in most individuals and should be avoided. One of the most reliable and safe solutions to constipation is small doses of magnesium throughout the day (Milk of Magnesia, 1-2 <u>teaspoons</u> (not tablespoons) three times daily). Stimulant laxatives should only be used occasionally or under the direction of a health care provider.

Another complimentary strategy recognizes that for certain individuals, carbohydrates commonly found in grain products feed abnormal bacteria in the colon. This strategy eliminates all grain products and other food sources that contain related carbohydrates in order to "starve out" undesirable bacteria. A special diet, referred to as the "Specific Carbohydrate Diet," defines the strategy. Details can be found in the book *Breaking the Vicious Cycle* by Elaine Gottschall, B.A., M.Sc. The diet has a following worldwide and is supported by several websites offering recipes and food suggestions. The diet often works, to which multitudes of sufferers can attest. *www.breakingtheviciouscycle.info*

Gastrointestinal dysfunction is common and mild symptoms often respond to dietary and lifestyle changes. Any out of the ordinary symptoms including vomiting, vomiting blood, passage of blood from the rectum, or any severe symptoms should be immediately reported to a healthcare provider.

Active

An active lifestyle is an important key to longevity.

CHAPTER 12

An Active Body

The top of this sand dune has the best view around. At approximately fifty feet above sea level, it is the highest natural point in the county. On a clear fall day you can make out the lighthouse at the cape several miles to the east. To the west are piers, condominiums, and beach houses. The inlet and port are in plain view, with boats and ships continually coming and going. Through them, it is easy to feel a connection with all of the rest of the world. This particular spot is a midway point on a path that I regularly hike during the cooler months of the year. It is a good spot from which to take in the whole world and take a break from it, all at the same time. The experience is certainly one of healthful defocusing.

The trail meanders along a narrow pathway around and over a couple of miles of sand dunes. The sand and the dunes provide more than just scenery. Unlike walking on pavement, the sand cushions stress on joints, but at the same time strengthens foot, calf and thigh muscles. The up and-down trek over dunes varies the level of exercise, without adding stress to the body. The trail is never quite the same. It changes from day to day and season to season, with the weather, the foliage, the tide, the birds, and the ocean. After a good workout, the beach offers a leisurely stroll back to the parking lot. If timing is right, this usually coincides with the sun setting on the horizon. The full route takes about an hour, and the last thing that I have on my mind is "having to exercise."

Regular vigorous physical activity is a necessity of good health, but the concept of "doing exercise" is a fairly new. Prior to the petroleum age, daily vigorous physical activity was simply part of life. Mobility, sustenance, and most everything else in life required physical labor. There was no reason to exercise. Today, obtaining food is a simple matter of driving to the store, and our jobs and lifestyles have become much more sedentary. Because physical labor is no longer a requirement for survival, doing enough physical activity to stay healthy is a matter of choice—a choice that seems to be difficult for many individuals.

When we start tallying up the reasons why we should be more physically active, the consequences of *not* being so become quite apparent. Vigorous physical activity is associated with an automatic increase in heart rate. The heart pumps harder to move more blood and carry more oxygen to active muscle fibers. Exercise causes blood vessels to dilate, or open up, allowing blood to flow more freely. The resulting increase in blood flow removes carbon dioxide and waste products from tissues. The rush of blood also washes out toxins and equilibrates hormones. In effect, exercise "blows out the pipes."

Vigorous physical activity mobilizes glucose and fat stores and allows the entry of glucose into cells even *without* insulin, an important factor in decreasing the incidence of insulin resistance and diabetes. The increased blood pressure and increased heart rate that occur with exercise are associated with chemicals that cause *dilation* of blood vessels, allowing blood to flow more freely. This is why regular exercise can alleviate hypertension, often without the use of drug therapy. The resulting increased blood flow reduces toxic buildup and atherosclerotic plaque formation, thus decreasing the risk of stroke and heart attack.

The benefits of exercise go beyond the physical. In our confrontation-filled world, stress stays "pent up" inside with no outlet. Exercise offers release that normalizes elevated levels of adrenaline. It is the normal endpoint of the "flight or fight" response. Regular exercise offers an outlet to diffuse and moderate stress in our lives.

With the benefits of physical activity being so obvious, you would think we would be stepping all over each other trying to get out and run around the block. Instead, it seems that most people have an aversion to exercise. Exercise, with the movement of muscles and ligaments over bones and joints, precipitates pain. Because it hurts to move, human nature would suggest that moving less is a good plan. This is actually the opposite of how it works. Regular exercise is associated with an *increase* in endorphins. These powerful chemicals not only decrease pain, but also are also associated with an increased sense of well-being. This is why drugs like morphine and heroin that mimic these natural chemicals are so profoundly addictive. The more regularly you exercise, the more liberally these chemicals are generated internally, and the better you feel.....naturally.

We would all be perpetual couch potatoes if it were not for natural pain-fighting endorphins floating around in our bodies. These "feel good" chemicals allow us to go about our normal daily activities without excessive discomfort, even though we have a baseline level of pain that is always there. Fortunately for most of us, the level is very low and easy to ignore, but it is there just the same. As we grow older the baseline pain level gradually creeps upward, and for individuals with conditions such as arthritis or fibromyalgia, the pain can be completely debilitating.

With exercise there is an initial increase in pain followed by a gradual, but corresponding increase in endorphins. It takes about 15 minutes for endorphin production to catch up. Many people never get past that first 15 minutes and relate exercise only to pain and discomfort. Why do something if it doesn't feel good? Sometimes in life you have to push past the pain to get the gain.

ADOPTING AN ACTIVE LIFESTYLE

A sedentary lifestyle is associated with a lower baseline level of endorphins, a higher baseline level of pain, a lower sense of well-being, and an aversion to exercise. An active lifestyle is, of course, associated with the opposite. How do we get from one to the other? Getting past that initial pain is challenging, and maintaining a comfortable flow of endorphins means doing some sort of exercise every day.

The focus of exercise should always be pleasure and never drudgery. The inevitable pain that comes with exercise can easily be diffused by the pleasurable aspects of exercise. Long ago I left behind the practice of doing exercise for the sake of doing exercise. *The key to making it work is raising the energy level of the body by becoming more active in every aspect of life. There are many ways to accomplish this goal, well beyond just working out at the gym.*

How you go about becoming physically active is a matter of personal choice. For my now adult children, a trip to a fitness center is an essential daily affair. They enjoy the social aspects and gain support from other people. For me, the thought of being confined to a stale-smelling room with forty other sweaty people working out on whining machines while televisions flash is next to torture. I like variety, space and solitude. Exercise is a part of my daily routine, but it varies from day to day. Whether hiking sand dunes, kite surfing when the wind is right, or biking to work or the grocery store, I can generally find something active to do.

Staying in good physical shape does not necessarily mean following a standard exercise routine. My wife regularly enjoys exercise classes offered at a local fitness center, but also achieves physical fitness through gardening and yard work. On a similar note, my parents, who are in good shape for being in their seventies, remain so by being physically active. They do much of their own home maintenance by choice and are constantly painting, repairing stutters, pulling up fence posts, and putting in new gardens. I have rarely known them to sit idle.

YOU HAVE TO START SOMEWHERE

Probably the biggest impediment to becoming more active is inactivity itself. Another common roadblock is excessive weight. Obesity is commonly associated with back, joint, and foot problems, aside from just having to move the extra mass. It takes perseverance, but the cycle can and must be broken. Overcoming this hurdle will undoubtedly involve a little pain, will probably cause some embarrassment, and at times will be boring. But if you persist, even before the weight comes off, stamina will improve, the pain will lessen, and a larger variety of activities will be possible. **Regular physical activity is essential for good health and losing weight.**

Start slowly with activities that are comfortable and safe, but make the most of them and try to do just a little more each day. Walking is good, but even better if up an incline like hills or sand dunes. Biking and swimming are easy on joints. Kayaking and rowing are affordable water sports that are excellent for including the upper body in a workout routine. **Any type of regular exercise raises the energy level of the body and burns more calories.**

Take advantage of supports for joint protection and special shoes to eliminate foot pain. A personal trainer or exercise counselor can be of real benefit. Trained individuals can guide you and keep you focused, even when you are ready to throw in the towel.

Being physically active should never seem like drudgery. It is truly one of the gifts of life. The reward of regular physical activity is being able to do things that you never thought possible. This is when exercise becomes fun.

It may lead you to develop a passion for some type of recreational activity.

It means not being just a spectator.

Beyond exercise just for the sake of exercising, it means taking on an active lifestyle.

It doesn't matter how you do it, but you need to work up a good sweat at least once a day...everyday!

Exercise Tips

Look for ways to be more active in everyday life. Go outside every chance you get. Make a habit of walking places instead of driving whenever you can. At the very least, park further from your destination and walk a bit more. Buy a bike! Take a hike! Join a fitness center and really use it. Become associated with active people. Spend your weekends being active. Build something. Create something. Grow something! Turn your yard into a garden. Working a shovel into the soil or even using a rake is great exercise.

Turn off the television! TV sucks the life out of you. It hypnotizes you into doing absolutely nothing – sometimes for hours. Obesity and television are intimately tied together. There are so many interesting things to do in life. Don't spend your time watching other people live their lives while yours is slipping by! If you have children, by all means limit their TV-watching, too.

Or use the television more wisely. Interactive computer games have come a long way since Pacman. The latest systems include wireless devices that detect body movements. Both motivational and instructional, these systems will guide you through a wide variety of complete workouts right in your own living room!

Learn a new sport. There are plenty of choices: tennis, hiking, basketball, swimming, walking, biking, racquetball, golf (without the cart, of course), mountain climbing, mountain biking, horseback riding, sailing, surfing, windsurfing, kite surfing, skiing, skating and many more. Take dance lessons. Go bowling. Becoming active recreationally and pursuing an activity to a certain level of skill builds confidence and positive feelings about life in general.

Get a pedometer. A pedometer is a simple device worn on the belt that measures the number of steps taken. Its use was originally popularized in Japan by Dr. Yoshiro Hatano as far back as 1965. Since then, many health groups have embraced his recommendation of 10,000 steps every day (about five miles) as an incentive to maintain fitness while going about daily routines. Pedometers can be purchased at sports equipment stores and most large discount stores.

Try out an exercise ball. For an under-$20 piece of exercise equipment, the Swedish exercise ball offers one of the best options for strengthening and toning muscles of the entire body. The ball can be used in a variety of ways, from stretching to total workouts. Used correctly, the exercise ball is excellent for back rehabilitation. The simple act of sitting on an exercise ball properly aligns the spine and tones the muscles of the body. Many people confined to sedentary jobs have found benefit from using an office ball in place of an office chair. Take an exercise ball and a couple of hand weights to work for brief workouts during the day.

Exercise balls can be purchased through the Internet or at your local fitness store. Make sure you get the correct size ball for your height. *Exercise Balls for Dummies* by LaReine Chabut is an outstanding resource for beginners.

Rev up your energy level during the day. That feeling of lethargy, loss of "pep," and lack of enthusiasm are signs of a decreased energy level. Sometimes low energy is a result of not eating properly during the day, not drinking enough liquids, or not sleeping well during the previous night. It can also have a physical cause, such as declining thyroid function. But often it is a result of everyday stress, monotony, and standing or sitting in the same position all day. Bringing your energy level up is actually easy to do. A couple of trips around the parking lot at a brisk pace can raise energy levels. Even ten minutes of stretching can help. The right kind of music can definitely have a positive effect. At the end of a long hard day, a 15- to 20-minute session of deep relaxation followed by 30 to 40 minutes of vigorous exercise can change your entire outlook on life.

An active lifestyle is not limited to the young or those who are already physically fit. I know of an individual who at age 92 is still passionate about tennis and stays in good physical condition for his age because of it. There are scores of handicapped individuals who are passionate about a recreational activity requiring physical fitness. Passion for physical activity is the distinguishing factor between exercising regularly and following an active lifestyle. Those who try to exercise regularly but don't enjoy it generally give it up. Those who adopt an active lifestyle often find it addictive!

Fitness centers can be a valuable resource and generally are worth the investment. Beyond being just basic exercise and recreational outlets, these centers offer a wide assortment of programs for improving health and physical fitness. Individuals with young children often find daycare and children's programs are available. Fitness centers can be extremely valuable not only in the pursuit of losing weight but also to become more health-oriented in general. Use the gym to remain motivated and stay in shape for other activities that you enjoy.

Don't let kids or your spouse be an impediment to being more active. Take them with you. Pick activities they can do also. Sports programs for children are great, but *don't just be a spectator.* Become involved in their activities and involve them in yours. You'll be a closer and happier family for it.

Take advantage of "free" exercise. Use physical labor to complete tasks that could otherwise require a machine or hiring someone. There are so many different ways to take advantage of this concept. Tilling and hoeing your own garden is a full body workout. Wash your own car. Walk or bike to work or to the store if you can. It requires a little extra planning and attention to the weather, but it can take some of the "ho hum" out of the day. Biking is excellent transportation and is easy on joints.

My sand dune hike lies within a state park that is only a ten-minute drive from my house. Search for places like this near where you live and whenever you travel. It adds a whole new dimension to the concept of staying in shape.

DOING EXERCISE RIGHT

Although the benefits of regular exercise are profound, there is a downside. Exercise causes wear and tear on joints and ligaments. The habit of performing a stretching routine prior to starting exercise reduces the potential for injury. Taking care of joints with proper supports in the event of strain or mishap is also very important. Practicing disciplines such as yoga keeps ligaments and muscles loose and improves balance. Proper nutrition keeps bones, ligaments, muscles, and joints healthy.

The sun can be intense. Protect your skin with clothing and/or moderate use of sunscreen before outdoor activities.

When pursuing recreation activities, set reasonable limits, follow good nutritional habits and drink plenty of water.

The intensity of exercise should be considered less important than the regularity of it.

There is always some discomfort when first beginning an exercise routine. In fact, the first 15 minutes of exercise is downright painful, even for those who exercise regularly. We call this the warm-up period. Breathing is faster and labored, muscles and joints are stiff, and it is just not pleasant. Gradually, breathing slows to a regular pace, everything kind of settles in, and it begins to actually feel pretty good. This "good feeling" is the result of endorphins and other chemicals being generated by exercise. Things stay like that for a while, and then as energy stores run low, fatigue begins to set in. The amount of time between warm up and exhaustion depends on the fitness level of the individual and the intensity of the activity. The sense of feeling good can last for hours after exercise is over.

When you take the step from being sedentary to becoming more active, the sense of feeling good associated with exercise may seem elusive at first, but don't give up: it will come, and your effort will be worthwhile.

HOW MUCH EXERCISE IS ENOUGH?

Official recommendations vary, but in actuality the correct answer is highly dependent on an individual's work requirements and lifestyle. Someone who regularly spends his or her days sitting behind a desk probably needs a good solid hour of formal exercise every single day, whereas a carpenter may need no formal exercise at all. Most of us probably fall somewhere in between. In my profession I may work inside an office, but find that I rarely sit still. Walking up and down halls, standing up, sitting down and constantly moving around is a necessity. Outside of the office I enjoy many types of recreation and am, in general, a very active person. This is the point.

Stay active. Never slow down. When you do is when you will grow old.
See your healthcare provider for personal guidelines before making the step toward an active lifestyle. Regular exercise is often an

important part of recovery from significant stress or illness, but the intensity and frequency of exercise should be adjusted according to the degree of debility. An overzealous exercise program in a stressed individual can be very disabling in itself and can worsen the individual's condition.

THE NEGATIVE SIDE OF EXERCISE

Weight-lifting can be beneficial, it but should not make up the majority of your exercise routine. The repetitive motion associated with weight-lifting is hard on ligaments and tendons. It is a common cause of tendonitis. If weight-lifting is part of your exercise routine, stay within reasonable limits and incorporate lifting along with other forms of exercise to achieve a whole body workout. Excessive weight-lifting can cause long term or permanent damage to ligaments and muscles. Set weights at a level that does not cause excessive strain. Gradually build up.

Bulking up may add to your looks, but will not add to your lifespan!

One concerning aspect of exercise is the increase in oxidative stress and toxin production caused by the elevation in metabolism for energy production. Antioxidants found in healthy diets help protect tissues from damage. Negative effects can be minimized by exercising regularly to stay in shape and building up to higher levels of exercise gradually. This is especially true if you have not exercised in a long time and/or have a history of atherosclerosis or other health problems.

Passions can sometimes carry exercise to an unhealthy extreme. Individuals who pursue competitions such as triathlons, long-distance running, and other extremes often place undue stress on the body. For some individuals, however, endurance training and extreme athleticism are an important part of getting the most out of life. Measures to protect the body during intense recreational activity include training, healthy diet, and brain synchrony exercises. Important dietary considerations include slow-release sources of glucose found in whole grains (especially barley and oats) and beans, healthy fats found in a variety of nuts and healthy sources of protein. Antioxidant protection should come from regular consumption of fresh vegetables, fresh berries, and citrus.

SYNCHRONY OF MIND AND BODY

In order to escape the tiger, the primitive man's brain and body had to be optimally synchronized. This state of being goes beyond simple physical activity. Often referred to as the "runner's high," it is associated with a feeling of being super-human. Many athletes find the feeling addictive and spend their lives pursuing it. Though this feeling can be achieved with any type of vigorous, focused physical activity, it is typically accentuated by the level of skill involved. Fortunately, you do not have to pursue extreme athleticism to enjoy the benefits.

DEFINING THE INTENSITY OF EXERCISE

Breathing defines how excited or relaxed we are at any given moment. Breathing is also the key to optimal exercise, because *how* you breathe during exercise very much influences the experience you will have.

When we're excited or anxious, we breathe through our mouths with quick, shallow breaths that only expand the upper portion of the lungs. Physical exertion, such as escaping a tiger, would be associated with the same type of breathing. Excitement causes release of adrenaline. Adrenaline mobilizes glucose stores for quick energy. Most people exercise in this fashion, huffing and puffing away, burning up glucose, but not fat.

During a time when I was monitoring blood glucose levels for self-interest, I happened to plop down on the couch in front of the TV (a rarity for me). The last hour of an intense Star Trek movie quickened my breathing and pumped up my pulse. Having not eaten anything for several hours, I decided it would be a great time to see how much adrenaline alone could affect blood glucose levels. A result of 150 was a surprise! I could have gotten it down by running around the block, but instead I simply relaxed and began doing deep-breathing exercises. Within 20 minutes my blood glucose was back down to 100!

When we are fully relaxed, we breathe through our noses. Breaths are slower and deeper and accompanied by expansion of the abdomen, as much as the chest. By using deep slow breathing during exercise, we send a message to the brain that we are relaxed. The body settles in for the long haul and fat is burned more readily, while glucose is conserved. Waste products are removed more efficiently. Stamina is increased. Synchronization of the body and mind happens naturally. Exercise becomes meditative and relaxing.

Many long-distance runners use this technique quite effectively. Try it the next time you exercise. Use mouth-breathing during warm-up and then gradually shift over to deeper and slower breathing. Deep breathing should expand the abdomen as well as the chest. Set your level of exercise to your ability to maintain deep breathing. When you lose the ability to hold on to deep slow breathing and have to revert to mouth-breathing, back off on the level of exercise for a couple of minutes until deep breathing can be resumed. In the beginning, the intensity of exercise may be lower than you are used to, but will gradually build back to normal. With this method you will find exercise to be more effective and enjoyable. Also, it is also hard to hurt yourself with exercise if you stick with deep abdominal breathing.

The concept of controlled breathing as a way to balance the body and mind has been around for ages. The ancient practices of tai chi, Qi gong (Chi gung), yoga, Pilates, and karate all use breathing to improve body fitness and, at the same time, synchronize the body and mind.

The mind and body are separate, but inseparable at the same time. Synchronization of the mind and body through exercise is a way to achieve this higher state of being necessary for optimal health.

Calm

Synchrony of the body and mind brings optimal health into focus.

CHAPTER 13

Left Brain / Right Brain

Though we think of a human as having a single brain, the thinking portion of the brain is actually divided in two halves. We refer to these halves as hemispheres. It is well known to most people that the left side of the brain controls the right side of the body and the right side of the brain controls the left side of the body, but it is seldom recognized that each of these hemispheres has independent functions that are unique.

The story behind our knowledge of independent right and left brain function is interesting. Patients with intractable seizures are sometimes treated with a surgical procedure in which the areas connecting the two hemispheres of the brain are severed completely. These patients have become known as "split-brain patients." After surgery, seizures typically resolve completely and amazingly these patients are able to return to being normal, functioning members of society—with no apparent disability. Unusual "quirks" can only elicited by specially designed experiments. These experiments offer insight as to how we cope with two brain halves that function quite differently.

In the most interesting of the experiments, a split-brain patient is placed in a booth specially designed to completely separate and isolate the left and right sides of the body. In the visual field of the left eye, the patient can plainly see a spoon and a knife lying on a table in front of them. A picture of a spoon is projected onto a screen, also on the left side. On the opposite side of the booth, in the right visual field, a spoon and knife are again present; identical to the ones on the opposite side, but a picture of a knife is projected onto the screen. Both eyes were able to see a spoon and a knife on a table, but the left eye is only able to see a spoon on the screen and the right eye is only able to see a knife on the screen. If asked to name the object on the screen, the patient would confidently reply, "knife." If asked to pick up the object displayed on the screen, the patient would always pick up a spoon.

Experiments with split-brain patients illustrate that we are all a product of two brains, each functioning independently, but both contributing to who we are. Some individuals tend to be more right-brained: more creative and more abstract in their approach to life, but oblivious to time. Most others tend to be more left-brained: punctual, preferring order and planning. Life is actually somewhere in the middle, with both sides being equally important. Learning to balance the functions of the brain is important for all of us.

The right hemisphere of the brain, controlling motor function on the left side of the body, is abstract, spatial, completely nonverbal, and has little sense of time. It is our source of creativity. The left side of the brain, responsible for controlling motor functions on the right side of the body, is concrete, analytical, verbal and very conscious of time. It allows us to deal with conflict.

In our modern world, the left brain is usually dominant; however, for most of human history, this was probably not the case. The mundane chore of collecting food required little in the way of left-brain function. Verbal skills took many thousands of years to develop and written language did not show up until very late in the course of human history. Even early cave drawings definitely came from the right brain. Time schedules were dictated only by the sun, the moon and the change in seasons. Thinking was mainly in terms of being aware of the surrounding natural world—very right-brained.

Early humans did need the analytical functions of the left brain, but not nearly as much as we do today. Left-brain functions were reserved mainly for dealing with conflict. Organizing a confrontation with the clan of humans over the hill for rights to the berry patch in the valley would have required left brain function. Calculating the number of sticks and rocks to have on hand and planning the route of attack would have been beyond the capacity of the right brain. Conflict was the ingredient that propelled us toward our world today.

Left-brained functions, though only used intermittently, were a necessity for dealing with conflict. When our prehistoric man came from around a rock to find himself face to face with a saber-toothed tiger, left-brain functions immediately came into play and the two halves of the brain blended synchronously to evaluate the threat. All within a fraction of a second, rapid analysis would define any possible tools available for defense and the best escape route.

This surge in left-brain activity came with a corresponding surge of adrenaline. Adrenaline is the hormone that prepares us for conflict. Physiologically, adrenaline causes increases in visual acuity, heart rate, blood vessel constriction, muscle tension and respiratory rate, all in preparation for fight or flight. Assuming he survived the encounter, our prehistoric man would gently ease back into berry-picking mode: his heart rate and respiratory rate would slow to normal. Gastrointestinal and immune system functions, which had been placed on hold during the brief incident, would also gradually resume.

Though conflict would seem undesirable, to be avoided if possible, the feeling that occurred when the primitive man escaped death at the jaws of the saber-toothed tiger must have been quite exhilarating. Very possibly he felt more alive at that particular moment than he felt at any other time in his life. The feeling that comes with brain synchrony drives many of us today. It is the feeling pursued by race-car drivers and high-level deal makers. It is often associated with conflict or risk.

At the height of intense conflict, the analytical ability of the brain functions at peak performance. Time seems to stand still. A heightened state of awareness occurs, representing optimal, synchronous functioning of the hemispheres of the brain.

Humans today are addicted to conflict. We seem to never get enough of the tiger. As a culture we thrive on it. When it doesn't come to us, we seek it out through interactions with other people, the news media, and the entertainment industry. We have, in essence, created a world of perpetual conflict, both real and imagined.

The state of perpetual conflict in which we exist today is very taxing. In the primitive man's world conflict was intermittent and could not be predicted; therefore, little anticipatory stress was associated with conflict. Today we are exposed to potential conflict around every turn. Conflict—perceived or real—causes us to constantly be on alert, always aware that the tiger is just around the corner. We worry about it incessantly. We exist in a state of perpetual adrenaline rush. In maintaining a perpetual state of alert, we are burning both ends of the candle at once. Our brain is constantly in the mode of dealing with conflict, creativity is suppressed, and normal maintenance functions of the body such as gastrointestinal function and immune functions are chronically placed on hold. Is it any wonder that insomnia, anxiety, hypertension, reflux and irritable bowel syndrome are the order of the day?

In addition to living in a world of perpetual conflict, we are constantly confronted with schedules, deadlines, and an almost unlimited amount of verbal and written information—all functions that depend exclusively on the left brain. One of the most obvious signs of left-brain dominance is the use of words. On a minute-by-minute basis, verbal skills are required for most everything we do. We write, talk and even think in words. Our left-brained world is a place of computers, cell phones, television monitors in every public place, schedules, deadlines and endless meetings. Being completely non-verbal, the right brain never gets a say and takes a backseat on every issue.

From an early age we are taught to use words to describe things, to be punctual, and to be very orderly. School and work tend to require a very verbal and analytical approach to life. Dawdling and daydreaming are always discouraged. *In essence, we are taught to turn off right-brain function.*

With right-brain function suppressed and the left brain always in control, the fundamental nature of brain synchrony is not possible and

the brain is left in a perpetually imbalanced state. The health costs of left-brain dominance are high: anxiety, insomnia, hyperactivity, attention deficit disorder, obsessive compulsive disorder, hypertension, gastrointestinal problems, and immune dysfunction are just some of the most obvious end-results.

To rectify the problem we must achieve balance. A state of total right-brain dominance is no more desirable than that of left-brain dominance. A right-brain dominant world would be free of stress, but at the same time mundane and monotonous. Stress is not all bad. Stress can be a positive motivating factor: it moves us to get things done. Without stress we would never have goals and aspirations. For optimal health and optimal life, we need to be able to use both sides of our brain equally, shifting from one side to the other, and synchronizing them when a challenging situation arises.

The first step in shifting away from left-brain dominant behavior is practicing exercises that allow right-brain activity to flourish. This is easier for some than others, as some individuals are more naturally right-brained, but anyone who makes an effort will receive benefit.

GETTING INTO "R-MODE"

Artists will often refer to being in "R-mode." I do a bit of drawing and can relate to this concept. If you try to draw a named object such as a face in the way you think a face should look, often the outcome is not very good. The left brain, as usual, is trying to run the show and dictates that the face should be drawn according to symbols it knows—a symbol for an eye, a symbol for a mouth, etc. The left brain is verbal and does not appreciate shapes, shades and patterns, so the symbols are not representative of the actual configuration of a face. Drawing in this fashion, with the right brain suppressed, is not only frustrating but often ends with poor results.

An effective method of teaching drawing involves changing the view of the object to be drawn such that the left brain is unable to identify the object. A picture of a face, once turned upside-down, becomes a complex mix of shapes and shades of light and dark. Now unrecognizable to the left brain, the right brain is finally allowed to take over. Sketching shapes and shades instead of defined objects becomes timeless and relaxing, and the outcome of the drawing is always more realistic. Drawing in R-mode is one of the most relaxing pastimes I have ever known.

Recognizing the potential to suppress the stress of the everyday world by drawing, I started looking for evidence of R-mode in other activities. I typically found it where nonverbal skills were required. Sailing, an activity I have done most of my life, is extremely relaxing. Thinking is in terms of sail trim, direction, speed and location relative to land and other objects. It is very nonverbal and very right-brained. At different times when I have taught sailing, I have found it difficult to explain the concepts in words because they are so right-brained. I used to think that sailing was relaxing just because of being physically away from everything, but I now understand it is because my left brain turns off from the moment I step on the boat.

Music can be approached from either a right-brained or a left-brained perspective. I spent several years trying to master the guitar by learning to read music and then interpreting the notes and rhythm from a sheet of paper onto the fingerboard and strings. This decidedly left-brained approach ended in frustrated failure. Had I approached the problem by listening to music and interpreting the music directly onto the frets and strings, I probably would have had a more relaxing and fulfilling experience. Many people learn better through right-brained experience and are often frustrated by the left-brained world. Very likely attention deficit disorder and hyperactivity have roots in this disequilibrium.

Mastering an instrument is not a necessary requirement for using music to achieve brain synchrony. The rhythm and beat of music predate verbal usage in human evolution by a wide margin. Listening to music is soothing and relaxing because it touches the right side of our brain as it calms the left. Of course, this is highly dependent on the type of music, as we each have our own taste. The right kind of music can help induce a state of brain synchrony during exercise, meditation, or even while at work.

Many focused nonverbal activities disengage left-brain function and at the same time disengage us from the oppressive worries of the world. Unfortunately, few of us have many opportunities to incorporate them into our daily lives. Learning some simple practices to use throughout the day can change your whole perspective on life.

TURNING OFF WORDS AND TURNING ON CREATIVITY

Using words is very left-brained. We tend to think in words. During the day we tend to get into a rhythm of thinking in words and then the words just keep coming. Turning off the flow is downright difficult, if not impossible. Breaking the cycle by incorporating right-brain activities into an average hectic day is not only relaxing but also increases productivity and creativity.

Recognizing how often you are thinking in words is not very difficult, as the left-brain pours out a continuous stream of words; the challenging part is turning it off. In our very verbal left-brained world, this practice must be cultivated. Throughout the day, make an effort to think without words. Pay attention to shapes of objects around you, especially in your peripheral vision, but without naming them.

As an exercise, pick a stationary object—an apple, ink pen, cell phone, or whatever is at hand. For several minutes, study the object intently. Without naming it or anything about it, appreciate its shape, the contours making up its margins, shades of light and dark on the surface, colors and reflections, and shadows surrounding the object. Appreciate dimensions within the object: length, width, depth and how they relate to one another. Close your eyes and imagine the object as if it were blank space, a void in the shape of the object. Notice that the flow of words, though not be turned off completely, have slowed considerably and you feel more relaxed and in control. Practice this exercise as often as you can throughout the day and especially when you are beginning to feel overwhelmed and uptight. You will be amazing at the relaxation and focus that result.

You can take the object exercise one step further by drawing the object. This type of drawing, called contour drawing, is a method of teaching drawing skills, but you do not need to draw well, or even have a desire to draw well, to receive benefit from this activity. Contour drawing is an exercise in pure right brain function that can be used by anyone, at any time, and in any place. A pen or a pencil and a scrap of paper are all the tools that are required.

The objective with this exercise is to reproduce the contours and shades of an object that is unidentifiable to the left brain on a sheet of paper in black and white. The "unidentifiable" part is accomplished by turning a picture upside-down or concentrating on the lines and shades of a very small part of the whole. As an example, you can use your opposite hand, held out in front of you, as the object to be drawn. Concentrate on the angles of the lines that make up the margins of your thumb, without identifying a "thumb." Draw in a continuous line very slowly, a millimeter at a time. Continue to draw all of the fingers. Pay attention more to the spaces between the fingers than the fingers themselves and mentally draw these shapes. Shade in light and dark *as you see them*, instead of how you think they should be.

Gradually you will find yourself slipping into R-mode. Time becomes less relevant and thought becomes more relaxed and focused. Completion of the drawing is irrelevant, as this is not the goal. The outcome of the drawing also does not matter, though you may find that you can draw better than you think! Having it framed is perfectly acceptable: I still have a small drawing of one of my son's tennis shoes from when he was ten years old.

Betty Edwards defined these concepts in *Drawing on the Right Side of the Brain*. I would highly recommend this classic book to anyone interested in learning how to draw and to anyone who just wants to learn how to relax.

DEFOCUSING

In his book *Open Focus*, Les Fehmi suggests that the anxiety and other ills associated with stress (most of the pain we experience in life) occur because our focus is too narrow, possibly as a result of left-brain dominance. He offers a solution of opening our focus to the surrounding world to diffuse concerns, defocus left-brained activity, and synchronize right- and left-brain function. Though his discussions and exercises are somewhat abstract, the principles are simple: broaden the focus of all of your senses and decrease left-brain dominance by the regular practice of exercises designed to encourage right-brain activity. Once mastered, these techniques are effective for treating everything from anxiety to chronic pain.

This experience is easy to achieve. Any place with an expansive view will suffice. It could be a mountain top in Colorado, a tall sand dune, or the roof of a tall building. Once there, take in the view with all of your senses. Pay attention to your peripheral vision as much as to the objects directly in front of you. The objects in the direct field should become secondary. Notice sounds and the direction from which they originate. Notice the smell and taste of the air. Notice the wind brushing against your skin. Notice the cool of the breeze on unprotected skin and the warmth of your toes inside your shoes. Notice an unavoidable calmness. Immerse yourself and become part of the scene.

You can actually have the same experience while sitting at your computer or reading a book. Purposefully, pay as much attention to the area surrounding the object in front of you as the object itself. Extend your concentration as far out into your peripheral vision as possible. Extend your peripheral vision to the point of being able to imagine objects behind you. Imagine any objects or shapes behind the computer screen as though the screen was not there at all. Notice any sounds and the direction from which they originate. Notice the smell and taste of the air around you. Notice any feelings such as anxiety or boredom and acknowledge them. Notice the feel of the keys against your fingers and any other sensations of touch. You have just taking a step towards synchronizing your brain and probably already feel more relaxed and comfortable than you did a few moments ago. Imagine how you would feel if you made the effort to do this several times every day. By expanding our focus we dilute out some of our dominant left-brained function and allow more right-brained activity, automatically creating balance.

Periodically breaking concentration completely can be a very effective way to decrease the tension associated with dominant left-brained thought. I call this "specific daydreaming." From an early age we are discouraged from daydreaming, and it is true that living in a fog is not conducive to getting ahead in the world, but diffusing our attention does seem to be a practical way to balance our brain function and ease tension.

These techniques are extremely effective for diffusing everyday stress, but must be practiced. The brain must be retrained to function in a different way. Throughout a busy day at work, take a moment or two to think *nonverbally* about some other place or activity. This type of thinking does not have to completely occupy your thoughts; it can be just enough to break your concentration and resynchronize the brain.

Though regular practice of right-brained activities would seem to be a waste of precious time (daydreaming, after all, is not to be condoned in our left-brained world), overall productivity generally increases. As the brain becomes more balanced and relaxed, creativity flourishes. Insurmountable obstacles seem less so. The flow of thoughts and words from the left brain gradually decrease and at the same time become less jumbled and more focused.

BRAIN SYNCHRONY

Every now and then, when we get things just right, the two halves of the brain become tuned harmoniously, and a state of heightened awareness occurs that can be associated with brain synchrony. It cannot be maintained perpetually, but we should be able to tap into whenever we desire. For the primitive man, it was being able to shift into brain synchrony by bringing in the analytical ability of the left brain when he confronted the tiger, thus preventing panic from ensuing. For us, it is shifting from a predominant left brained existence by incorporating right brain activities. The feeling of brain synchrony is like none other.

- *It is the classic runner's high.*

- *It is when we are at the top of our game and on top of the world.*

- *It is a feeling of confidence and calmness, even under the most adverse of situations.*

- *It is being aware of everything around you, and beyond.*

- *It may be the feeling of true happiness.*

- *It is often the answer to depression and anxiety.*

- *It is a powerful force of healing.*

- *It is the state of being that many seek through meditation.*

- *It is the place where we go just before falling into blissful sleep.*

- *It is the feeling that many pursue through pharmaceuticals and illicit drugs, but quickly find that this shortcut is short-lived and fades into the misery of withdrawal and addiction.*

The state of brain synchrony can be measured by a device called an EEG machine. An electro-encephalogram (EEG) is a tool that measures the electrical activity of the brain. This activity is quite dynamic and changes from minute to minute and even from second to second. Patterns of brain wave activity reflect the particular state of awareness an individual may be experiencing at any given moment.

The erratic and irregular waves produced by a brain functioning as left-brain dominant are termed *beta waves.* Most of us exist in this less- than-desirable state on a daily basis. When the two sides of the brain are synchronized, mental acuity and brain performance are optimal. This wave is represented by a smooth and regular wave called an *alpha wave.* An alpha pattern is where we would like to be more of the time than we actually are. Deep meditation causes further smoothing of the wave into a *theta wave* and deep sleep rounds out the pattern even further into a *delta wave.*

Brain synchrony not only bodes well for mental performance and a strong sense of well-being (even during life's most extenuating circumstances), but also relates to good health in general. Production of alpha, theta, and delta waves is associated with optimal healing and optimal immune function. Regular practice of right-brained exercises, relaxation techniques, and meditation all promote optimal healing.

Just as left-brained desynchrony is a learned behavior (many bad habits are learned behaviors), consistent production of alpha waves, associated with brain synchrony, is also a learned behavior. Breaking old habits and learning new ones does take some effort, but anyone willing to practice can achieve this goal. Consistently being able to achieve a state of brain synchrony can be accelerated through a discipline called biofeedback.

There are different modalities for conducting biofeedback. An instrument called an EMG can be used to measure muscle tension, allowing the patient to more effectively relax muscle groups. A simple thermometer can be used to measure finger temperature, providing feedback on adrenaline release, which causes constriction of blood vessels and the classic cold hands of anxiety. In one of the most effective forms of biofeedback, brain waves can be measured with an EEG machine, allowing the patient to learn brain synchrony directly. This is referred to as neuro-biofeedback.

As we progress further into the electronic age, biofeedback will become more available on an individual basis. Once relegated to a clinical or laboratory setting, inexpensive instruments of different types are becoming available for "home" biofeedback. At some point in time, biofeedback may become the preferred treatment for any stress-related disorder.

With or without the advantage of biofeedback training, brain synchrony exercises are effective for treatment of almost any stress-related disorder, with positive benefit noted for anxiety, attention deficit disorder, hypertension, reflux, irritable bowel syndrome, migraines, insomnia, and menopausal symptoms. Brain synchrony is also an avenue toward higher brain performance in general. Whether your goal is improved job performance, heightened athletic ability, or just feeling more in tune with the world, the concept of synchrony of the body and mind should be explored.

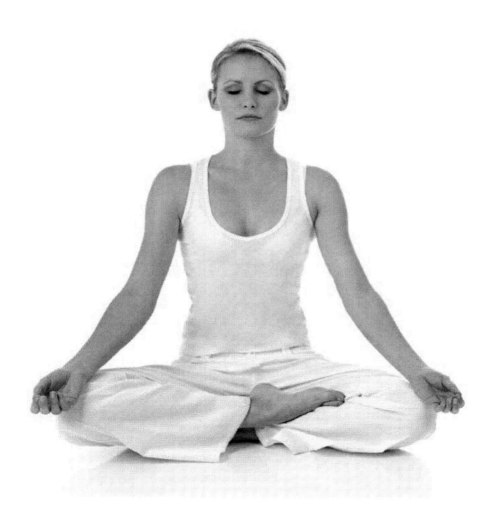

VITAL PLAN

CHAPTER 14

A Calm Mind

It is possible to seemingly do everything right from a health point of view and still be unhealthy. Even with a healthy diet, regular exercise and avoidance of toxins, without the last (and most difficult-to-achieve) piece of the puzzle in place, good health is not assured. In modern society, emotional stress is one of the largest threats we face. Learning effective tools for minimizing and managing stress is an absolute and essential part of maintaining good health.

The feeling of being "stressed out" is something that we have all experienced and something that some individuals live with every day. Being overly stressed is a symptom of not having control of life's situations, of the behavior of others, of work schedules, and of time itself. Sometimes this feeling is real and sometimes it is the way we perceive life to be. This sense of loss of control contributes to a feeling of hopelessness, the root of depression. Anxiety and depression rob the body of vital energy. Emotional stress affects the hormone systems of the body, suppresses the immune system, and in doing so increases the risk of almost every known disease.

On a biochemical level, emotional stress affects hormone release by the adrenal glands. We actually have two adrenal glands, located at the top of each of our kidneys. The middle portion of the gland secretes the hormone epinephrine, better known as "adrenaline." Adrenaline is the hormone that raises our heart rate, heightens our senses, quickens our reflexes, and makes us more alert when we are confronted with a threat. A surge of adrenaline can be life-saving when we are confronted with emergencies. It was the driving force that often kept our primitive man alive when he was confronted by a saber-toothed tiger.

The outer portion of the adrenal gland produces several hormones, with the most important one being cortisol. Cortisol is the "life giving" hormone, for without it we would quickly perish. Cortisol prepares the systems of the body for stress. During times of emotional stress or perceived threat, we secrete more cortisol so the systems of our body will be ready to meet the challenge. Increased cortisol shifts the resources of the body away from everyday concerns such as digesting food and repairing cumulative damage toward handling any immediate threat. **When we have the perception that a threat is always imminent, cortisol secretion remains higher than normal.**

Some stress is a normal part of life and the hormones adrenaline and cortisol allow us to deal quite well with this everyday stress. Stress only becomes a problem when it is overwhelming and, in particular, chronic. Maintaining persistently elevated levels of adrenaline and cortisol "burns both ends of the candle at once," causing us to age faster and have a higher susceptibility to disease. In shifting the resources of the body away from everyday maintenance and repair, cumulative damage starts to add up and eventually the body starts to deteriorate.

Chronically high levels of cortisol and adrenaline adversely affect all of the hormone systems of the body including the other adrenal hormones controlling fluid balances, the chemical messengers controlling the neurological system, the messengers and hormones of the immune system, the hormones of the gastrointestinal system, and the reproductive hormones. In addition, since people often respond to stress by overeating, there is the added problem of excessive consumption of glucose with associated increased insulin secretion. What a mess! Expect a forecast of high blood pressure, fluctuating blood glucose levels with episodes of hypoglycemia, agitation and irritability, insomnia, gastrointestinal problems, increased risk of heart attack and stroke, infertility, abnormal periods, allergy symptoms and/or many other conditions.

Adrenaline and cortisol secretion are under direct control of the higher brain by way of the HPA axis and autonomic nervous system (see Chapter 4). Schedules, verbal interactions and tedious analytical tasks—all functions of the left hemisphere of the brain—are the primary driving forces behind stress intolerance. A concerted effort to shift behavior toward right-brain function is one way of alleviating the perception of stress.

Regularly incorporating right-brain exercises into daily life reduces the perception of being overly stressed and allows stress to be a motivating factor instead of a detriment.

ANXIETY

Adrenaline is useful when it comes in controlled spurts. Adrenaline propels us toward the level of brain synchrony that allows us to deal with everyday stress. But often the stresses of life surpass everyday worries and concerns. Job changes, financial worries, challenges with raising children, personal illness, illnesses of loved ones and negative interactions with other people can be overwhelming. When the stress of life builds to the point of becoming oppressive, anxiety is the result. You can feel it building like a storm. Adrenaline levels start to rise—first as a small cloud, then a squall, and sometimes on to a raging tempest, difficult to control. Once established, it can take days or even weeks to dissipate.

The storm of anxiety depletes the calming neurotransmitters of the brain, leaving the nervous system in an agitated state. Anger, fear, irritability, worry and poor concentration are some of the most typical symptoms of anxiety. Physical manifestations of anxiety can often include gastrointestinal symptoms, chest pain, palpitations and difficulty breathing. Once a person becomes susceptible to anxiety, spontaneous episodes of anxiety known as panic attacks can occur. Sleep disturbances are often associated with anxiety, as dysfunctional fluctuations of adrenaline and cortisol keep the mind abnormally alert.

Recognizing when adrenaline production is getting out of control and defusing the storm before it starts to build are keys to controlling anxiety.

INSOMNIA

Approximately 25-50% of people suffer from insomnia at some point in their lives. Insomnia is not actually a disease, but a symptom of disease. Insomnia can have many causes. For some people it is chronic pain, for others it is a periodic disruption of normal breathing at night that we call "sleep apnea." Many medications cause disruption of sleep. Food allergies and gastrointestinal dysfunction can cause insomnia. Most commonly, though, it is a reaction to chronic stress, causing disruptions in the normal hormonal and neurotransmitter pathways associated with sleep.

The same chemicals that keep us calm during the day also keep us asleep at night. The main calming neurotransmitter of the brain is gamma amino butyric acid, called GABA for short. There are different GABA receptors in the brain; some keep us calm but awake during the day and others maintain sleep at night. The exact mechanism by which all this happens is not completely understood; in simple terms, it appears that stress, anxiety, worry and even pain "use up" GABA and leave the brain in an excited and sometimes agitated state. An alert mind is associated with increased adrenaline secretion. Cortisol follows adrenaline and keeps the brain alert as well. A vicious, self-perpetuating cycle is created. Sleep is next to impossible in states of increased adrenaline and cortisol production.

There does seem to be a genetic predisposition for insomnia. Perhaps the distant ancestors of today's poor sleepers were the easily-roused survivors who alerted the others when danger was near. In our hyper-stimulated world, however, being such a light sleeper can become an unhealthy aggravation. Stressful lifestyles, stimulants such as caffeine, artificial lighting, computers, televisions, and odd work schedules are just some of the contributors to disruption of the normal hormones involved with sleep. On top of it all, it seems to worsen as we age.

For me, insomnia has always been the most obvious outward manifestation of stress. By age 45, burning both ends of the candle balancing a busy obstetrical practice with the rest of life caught up with me. Even with improved dietary habits and regular exercise, my health slowly began to deteriorate. At first I turned to the world of conventional medicine for help, but quickly found that my body and synthetic medicines are not compatible. (Retrospectively, there is little doubt that medical therapy hindered and prolonged recovery.) Ultimately, I took matters into my own hands and set forth on a self-directed course of rehabilitative therapy. A complete (and more sensible) lifestyle change, carefully chosen natural therapies, and years of practicing relaxation techniques gradually brought me back to a level of normal health and a regular good night's sleep.

The nature of sleep is very complex. For most mammals, cycles of sleep are obviously tied to cycles of night and day, but they are also a product of how a certain animal evolved. Dolphins, horses, rabbits, and tigers all have very different sleep cycles from those of humans. In most animals, episodes of deep sleep are necessary to allow the resources of the body to be focused totally on healing.

In humans there are four different stages of sleep as defined by brain wave patterns and another type of sleep, defined by rapid eye movements, that we call "REM" sleep. In terms analogous to a computer, REM sleep is the time when we put all of our files back in order for the next day. You can think of dreams as your screen saver. Stages one and two are lighter stages of sleep. Healing occurs most intensely when people are in stages three and four of sleep, at which point they are very hard to arouse. We tend to spend less and less time in stages three and four as we age.

Humans typically go in and out of the different cycles of sleep throughout the night, spending only a few hours in stages three and four sleep during an eight-hour rest period. In our world today this would seem to be quite inefficient. Certainly diving directly into three or four hours of intense deep sleep and being done with it would be practical, but this is not how we evolved. In distant times, becoming almost comatose for several hours at a time would have been an almost certain invitation to be eaten by something large; for survival purposes we learned to catch short intervals of deep sleep here and there. This seemingly inefficient sleep pattern is the one that we must live with today.

The good news is that insomnia really is just a symptom and will resolve if all of the causes are removed. Imbalances in neurotransmitters rectify themselves if given the right opportunity. Sometimes proper diagnosis involves a trip to a sleep clinic for disorders like sleep apnea, restless legs syndrome or narcolepsy, but for the everyday type of insomnia most common in our fast-paced world, the treatment is a matter of normalizing hyper-stimulated adrenal and nervous system functions. Interestingly, the key to a good night's sleep hinges mainly on how effectively we manage stress during the day.

A good night's sleep is an essential component of good health. Sleep is the time when the operating systems of the body are being fine-tuned, general maintenance functions are being performed and the immune system is functioning at peak level. Without sleep, all systems of the body suffer and the incidence of disease increases.

CHRONIC FATIGUE

When you push the stress button hard enough or for long enough, it all adds up. This situation can occur at any age, but is more common after forty. With chronic or excessive stress, adrenaline keeps pushing the body, even when it cannot be pushed any further; however, at some point, the resources of the body become taxed to the extent that a normal response to stress is impossible. Having lost the ability to keep up, the normal rhythmic fluctuations of cortisol become dysfunctional. Without normal cortisol secretion, the body loses the ability to appropriately manage day-to-day functions.

When fatigue regularly reaches a certain level it becomes known as chronic fatigue syndrome. Though fatigue is the most obvious symptom, chronic infections, anxiety, sleep disturbances, weakness and depression are typical. When accompanied by muscle and ligament pain, the condition is called fibromyalgia. Usually there is an inciting factor such as traumatic physical stress, prolonged emotional stress, severe work stress, or possibly a viral or bacterial illness; nevertheless, once established, adrenal dysfunction is always part of the picture. All systems of the body are adversely affected, including (and especially) the immune system. Many chronic conditions including pain syndromes and autoimmune diseases may be related to this same mechanism.

Chronic fatigue is, as much as anything else, a manifestation of imbalances within the entire hypothalamic-pituitary-adrenal axis. As you remember from Chapter 4, the HPA axis allows us to respond to change. Without this balance, all systems in the body are affected. Adrenal dysfunction and fatigue always go hand in hand. Thyroid dysfunction is commonly associated with chronic fatigue. Chronic fatigue is common in menopausal females. Effective therapy for chronic fatigue always includes support of hormonal function and reducing all stress factors, such that normal balance can return to all functional systems of the body.

DEPRESSION

Mood is normally a pendulum swing between happy and sad, a natural reflection of life's ups and downs. Mood becomes depression when life's pendulum becomes hung on the down side. This happens to all of us from time to time, with some people being more susceptible to depression than others. The downside of life is often a matter of perception: is the glass half full or half empty?

Depression can be defined in chemical terms. Sadness, in reaction to life's events, affects the balance of neurotransmitters within the brain. Many neurotransmitters are involved, but *serotonin*, the so-called "mood hormone," is the most often considered. Hormone imbalances associated with depression can usually be related to a specific cause—intense or prolonged anxiety, exhaustion from severe insomnia, a tragic occurrence, prolonged illness or hormonal changes associated with menopause, for instance—but occasionally depression seems to happen even in the absence of such inciting factors.

The causes of depression may be present but not readily obvious. Diets high in sugar and processed starch are associated with higher rates of depression. It is also noteworthy that toxins produced by abnormal strains of bacteria in the GI tract have shown ties to depression. Exposure to toxins in general may adversely affect the hormone systems of body enough to contribute to depression.

Some individuals have a genetic predisposition toward depression and are therefore more apt to feel depressed even in the absence of inciting factors. For them, the glass is always half empty. Genes cannot be altered and this is a situation where properly administered medicinal therapy can be life-changing. Another situation where pharmaceutical therapy may be indicated is in the case of individuals having wider "pendulum swings" than average. Referred to as manic-depression or bipolar disorder, this condition is also a function of genetic susceptibility.

Regular exercise, avoidance of processed foods, appropriate counseling and support groups are as important as drug therapy for management of depression.

HORMONE-DRIVEN STRESS INTOLERANCE

The normal cyclic reproductive cycle that a woman experiences each and every month is closely tied to all other functions in the body. Dysfunction or abnormal fluctuations of hormones within this cycle can cause stress intolerance, fatigue, mood changes, anxiety, depression and swelling, a collection of symptoms commonly known as premenstrual syndrome. Though some individuals do seem to have a genetic predisposition, symptoms are often tied to poor nutrition, exposure to hormonal active toxins, poor sleep habits and poor stress management skills. Improvements in health habits and stress modification are often associated with resolution of symptoms.

Cessation of reproductive function, referred to as menopause, is a natural part of a woman's life, but the hormonal changes that occur during and leading up to menopause can be the trigger for stress intolerance, anxiety, insomnia, fatigue, depression, or all of the above at the same time. Most of the symptoms will pass with time, but appropriately administered hormone therapy or alternative therapies can ease symptoms and help to save a job, a relationship, or even a life.

Though less well defined, a gradual decrease in normal male reproductive hormones with age can be associated with symptoms fatigue, stress intolerance and mood changes. Poor nutrition, exposure to hormonally active toxins, poor sleep habits and poor stress management skills can often be defined as inciting factors. Hormone function often normalizes along with symptoms when these inciting factors are removed.

DEFUSING EVERYDAY STRESS

The anticipation of stress is usually worse than stress itself. To get rid of stress, or at least the perception of it, we must periodically turn-off the very verbal, analytical and time-conscious left brain (as was discussed in Chapter 12). In doing so, we connect with the all-important hormone regulatory system in a calming way. Adrenaline production is decreased and the rhythms of cortisol secretion are normalized.

Turning off the left side of the brain is not necessarily an easy task in our very left-brain dominant world. Effectively suppressing the left brain and allowing right-brain functions to flourish takes practice and effort, but there is a reward: reconnecting with the creative, calmer side of your mind not only reduces stress but also balances life and allows you to reach your full potential as a human being.

Wandering off into the right side of your brain every now and then is a perfectly acceptable way of achieving lasting mental health. Some people do it in a big way, such as by casting off for a three-year cruise around the world, but such drastic steps are rarely necessary. Many hobbies (drawing, needlepoint, woodworking, fishing, sailing and gardening are just a few examples) require skills that originate from the right side of the brain.

If you do not have a hobby, consider adopting one. If you already have a hobby, consider making it a more prominent part of your life.

There are many different ways of dealing with stress, from simple to complex. Any of the right-brained exercises found in Chapter 12 can be beneficial. Your approach to life—how you deal with people and situations—does matter, and a positive attitude is more important than anything else. Though we cannot control all of life's variables, we do have choices. Choices that reduce personal stress have the potential to improve not only our own lives but also the lives of everyone around us.

Listen to your body. The tension associated with the building storm of stress and anxiety can rise rapidly. Recognizing the early signs of tension is the first step in learning how to defuse stress.

RELEASING MUSCLE TENSION

One of the most obvious effects of built-up stress is muscle tension. Whether due to an injury or just from walking outside on an extra cold day, we all tend to brace against pain by reflexively tightening up the muscles of the back, neck, and shoulders and breathing in a rapid, shallow fashion. We brace against the building discomfort of stress in the same way, except that muscle tension becomes a normal state of being instead of just a transient phenomenon. Chronic back, neck, and shoulder pain, as well as tension headaches, can be the result of built-up muscle tension.

Do a tension assessment. At any given moment you are probably more tense than you realize. Learn to recognize the feeling of your body bracing against stress.

How is your breathing? Is it shallow and quick or deep and slow? Are you breathing just within the upper part of your chest or down into the deeper chest and abdomen?

How cold are your hands and feet? Adrenaline causes constriction of peripheral blood vessels. A relaxed state is associated with warm feet and hands.

What is your focus of attention—intensely narrow or more diffuse?

How tense are the muscles of the shoulders and neck?

Every time you feel stress building, resist the urge to tighten up.

As much as an uptight posture is a sign of tension, maintenance of a relaxed posture makes it almost impossible to be uptight.

Relax your abdomen and roll back your shoulders. Loosen them up and let them fall until limp. Breathing will automatically slow down and become deeper.

Remind yourself a hundred times a day if necessary:
  Relax the shoulders and breathe deeply.

This simple little exercise is amazingly effective. Every time you remind yourself to relax the shoulders, also get in the habit of taking three deep breaths through the lower part of your abdomen. Not only will you feel more relaxed but you will also ward off tension headaches and neck pain.

Movement is another effective method of diffusing tension. If you have a sedentary job, do not sit in one place any more than necessary. Move around. Walk everywhere you can. During a lunch break, make a habit of going for a walk or doing some kind of physical activity. Activity gets blood flowing and diffuses the focus of concentration. Try an exercise ball (see Chapter 13).

Stretching is an excellent way to diffuse stress and relieve tension. The discipline of yoga is the most commonly practiced form of stretching found today. Though formal classes are very beneficial for beginners, the stretching poses can be done nearly anywhere. Once several basic poses are learned, they can be incorporated into daily routines.

ESCAPE FROM THE STORM

Much of stress has more to do with how we <u>perceive</u> the world to be than how it actually is.

There are people who have endured greater stress than you or I will ever know and lived to tell about it.

Life is synonymous with challenge and conflict. How we <u>deal</u> with challenge and conflict involves learned behaviors. As much as life teaches us to be anxious, we can also learn to be calm, even in the face of great adversity.

Even the most anxious individual has moments of absolute calmness. Learning how to cultivate moments of calmness in the face of stress is an essential skill for overcoming anxiety and gaining control over stressful situations. Individuals who regularly practice relaxation techniques handle any type of stress better.

The issue of overcoming stress and anxiety is about regaining control. Sometimes even the perception of regaining control is enough to defuse stress and anxiety. Learning effective tools for diffusing stress is essential for maintaining good health.

Moments of complete calmness interspersed throughout the day are important not only for reducing anxiety but also for regaining control of life. Methods for mastering spontaneous relaxation have been around for most of eternity. Meditation, yoga, and prayer are time-tested activities that all induce a relaxed state. Newer and more defined techniques such as progressive relaxation, autogenics, self-hypnosis, and brain synchrony exercises focus specifically on relaxation.

The common denominator for all relaxation techniques lies in producing a shift from the analytical thought of the left brain to the more abstract thought processes of the right brain. The most notable feature of an over-excited mind is the constant stream of verbal thought. All effective relaxation techniques block or slow the flow of verbal thought from the left brain. In doing so, the body relaxes and adrenaline levels decrease. The functions of the body normalize and the healing potential of the body increases. Attention to breathing is a good place to start this process.

LEARNING HOW TO BREATHE

Attention to breathing synchronizes many of the functions of the body. Our breath flows as life-giving oxygen into the blood, which carries it to every part of the body, where it provides a critical part of energy production in cells.

The first step in learning how to relax spontaneously is learning controlled breathing. Breathing is unique in that it is an "autonomic" or automatic response that can also be controlled with voluntary actions. When we control our breathing it ties into other autonomic responses. Slowing the rate of breathing is associated with a decreased heart rate, decreased blood pressure, and—very importantly—decreased adrenaline levels. Slowed breathing also is associated with increased production of endorphins, those wonderful internal chemicals that improve our sense of well-being.

Most of us breathe with our chest muscles. The more uptight we are, the shorter and shallower the breath becomes, and the more tension there is in the shoulders and neck. When relaxed, we use abdominal breathing: instead of using the chest wall muscles, we are then using mainly the diaphragm.

Observe this by first lying comfortably on your back. Control and slow your breathing to an easy rhythm. Place one hand on the abdomen, close to the belly button. As you breathe, try to keep the chest wall still and pull air into the lungs by expanding the abdominal muscles. Your hand should rise and fall with each breath. Breathing should be done through the nose, not through the mouth. Inhalations and exhalations should be equal.

It takes a little practice. Relaxation happens quickly, even after only a few minutes. Focused concentration on breathing by itself is a simple and profoundly effective relaxation technique that can be done nearly anytime you have a few minutes—while waiting at a stoplight, during a break at the office, or while waiting for water to boil.

Try this simple breathing exercise. Using abdominal breathing, try to extend your breath for as long as possible without holding your breath. Inspiration and expiration should be equal. At first attempts, your inspiration and expiration will be about 5-7 seconds each, but your goal is to extend each to 15 seconds, resulting in only 2 complete breaths in one minute. Don't strain. Make it easy and comfortable. Work up to 15 seconds slowly. You can practice this one anywhere, even at a stoplight.

Another simple breathing exercise is sequential count-to-ten. Using abdominal breathing of normal length, begin counting each breath. Count first to up to 2 and then start over, 1-2-3. Continue with 1-2-3-4, and so forth, up to the sequence 1-10. It takes more concentration than you can imagine. Completion of two sequences of 10 often results in deep relaxation with lowered pulse rate and normalized blood pressure. This is also a great exercise to improve focus.

RELAXING THE BODY

We tend to take the functions of the body for granted. Becoming more attuned to the functions of the body is a very important step in synchrony of the body and mind. Awareness of muscle tension and learning how to relax the different muscle groups of the body is a way to monitor how the body is doing overall. Assessing muscle tension and responding by relaxing muscles can be done on a limited basis throughout the day. Progressive muscle relaxation, a formal technique, requires more time but is a powerful tool for health.

The basic goal of this technique is complete relaxation of each of the muscle groups in the body. Start in a supine position (i.e., on your back) with support of the head and legs. Establish controlled, relaxed abdominal breathing. Progressively concentrate on each area of the body independently. Work up from the feet to the calves to the thighs, hips, back, and abdomen. Progress to the chest, shoulders, upper arms, lower arms, and then finally to the hands. Don't forget the neck, ears, face, and cheeks. Last of all, imagine your forehead becoming as smooth and flat as possible. It is helpful to imagine a feeling of warmth and heaviness. This exercise can also be done in a relaxed standing position, working from the top of the head down to the feet.

If relaxing muscles seems difficult or if you are particularly uptight and tense, another technique makes use of progressive tightening of each of the muscle groups independently—as tightly as possible—and then relaxing. In the beginning, it may be helpful to purchase an audio tape or CD on progressive relaxation. With practice, muscle relaxation will become almost spontaneous.

RELAXING THE MIND

Now that the body is relaxed, it's time to work on relaxing the mind. The practice of calming the mind is most often referred to as meditation.

Meditation is an oasis that is always there, always within reach, but sometimes hard to grasp. It can free you of worry and the constant stream of intruding thoughts. It does not have to involve odd positions, weird music, or chanting. It can be anything you want it to be.

There are a number of different forms of meditation and many different perspectives on how to meditate. There is nothing magical or mystical about meditation. Simple daydreaming is a form of meditation. The most intense form of meditation is when all attention is focused on nothing. Clearing the mind of *all* thoughts, however, is extremely difficult and requires a great amount of practice. Most of us need to focus our attention on something. This can really be anything: our breathing, counting sheep, a candle flame, a monotonous sound, a mental image, or even a thought. Again, the common denominator is slowing or stopping the flow of words, such that a shift from left-brain dominance to right brain function occurs.

The most frustrating part of meditation, especially for beginners, is making the shift happen and knowing when it occurs. One of the more effortless ways to achieve this goal is through the techniques of "Open Focus" as described by Dr. Les Fehmi. Dr. Fehmi is one of early pioneers of neuro-biofeedback; with thirty years of experience in practice and research, he has refined these techniques quite well. They can be discovered through his book *Open Focus Brain*. The book comes with a CD demonstrating the techniques. Not only are these methods effective, but, more importantly, they are easy to master.

Open focus is a good place to start for many people, but it should be noted that there are many forms of meditation or spontaneous relaxation, and you have to find the one that works best for you. Meditation can involve formal techniques, but it also can be very informal. Monotonous activities or tasks, such as knitting or woodworking, can consume the mind enough to push unwanted thoughts away and encourage a relaxed state of mind. Simply focusing on something calming is also effective. A favorite CD of mine is of ocean waves crashing on a California beach. It's easy to focus on the waves and imagine actually being there.

During meditation and relaxation, outside thoughts often try to intrude. How much they intrude depends on the complexity of life and the stress level at that particular time. When thoughts intrude, recognize them, gently push them away or just notice them without allowing them to be the dominant thought, and refocus on the topic of concentration. If thoughts are overwhelming, stop, get up, and walk around. Get a snack or a drink and then start all over again.

THE REGULAR PRACTICE OF MEDITATION

Sages, monks and some spiritual leaders may meditate for five hours every day, but their goals are very different from yours and mine. From a health point of view, preventing excessive flow of adrenaline is our main objective. Some days, life is not very challenging and the need to meditate may not be there at all. On other, more stressful days we may desperately need a full five hours of meditation. Here lies the rub: on the most stressful days we tend to have the least time to step away. This is why incorporation of spontaneous relaxation into our daily lives and the regular practice of meditation are so important.

In an overly stressful world, individuals with any significant anxiety maintain a hypersensitive adrenal gland. Even the thought of a stressful situation sends adrenaline levels soaring. For health and happiness, this over-active gland needs to be tamed and the most positive way to do it is through regularly practiced meditation or self-relaxation. As with any skill, the body and mind respond to training. With training, the gland becomes less hypersensitive and stressful situations are better-tolerated.

Training means daily practice. It may require getting help from others. This can be in the form of audio/video resources or it can be direct training from an experienced individual. At the very least, make a pledge to sit quietly and simply focus on breathing for 10 minutes two times daily for eight weeks. Don't try too hard. Let it come naturally. If you stay with it, this simple pledge will change your life. As meditation becomes more comforting and comfortable, connecting with your inner self will become an essential part of daily life.

RESOURCES FOR MEDITATION

Meditation should be comfortable and something to look forward to. It should not be thought of as a chore and should not have special requirements for time and place. Peace and quiet are helpful, but not essential; I have had some success with meditation in the middle of a busy airport.

Position is also less important than some sources would have you think. The classic "lotus" position works well for some people, but any sitting or lying position is acceptable. This can be in a lounge chair, lying on the floor, lying in bed, or even sitting on your porch steps.—anywhere that is comfortable for you. Remember, the primary purpose of meditation is relieving stress and therefore it should not be a stressful experience.

There are many excellent resources in book, CD and DVD formats for help in mastering these techniques. An Internet search for "spontaneous relaxation" or "meditation" will bring up a plethora of choices. These guided sessions will help your practice become more regular and effective. Another very useful and novel adjunct is special music with brain waves super-imposed. This work was pioneered by Dr Jeffrey Thompson and can be readily found on the Internet. He has composed a variety of different formats for encouraging concentration, meditation, and even sleep. I have found them to be very effective tools and use them regularly to arrive at a deeper state of relaxation more quickly. An MP3 player is another helpful tool. A large number of relaxation CD's can be loaded into these portable devices.

Find yourself a special place.

The concept of a special place is an important one. For some it is an icy mountain top in Patagonia; for others, it is a quiet garden in the back corner of a yard. Generally it is a place of peace and solitude, away from everything and everyone. You can have more than one. Going there frequently can help maintain your sanity even during stressful times. Traveling to special places can be a lot of fun also. Some people spend entire vacations seeking out special places in natural areas such as our national parks. Sometimes just knowing that these places exist is enough to give you a sense of peace. A special place can be the object of meditation even if you cannot go there.

Why are gurus always pictured sitting on a mountain top? The symbolism is not lost on those who meditate regularly. The mountaintop represents being above all worry and stress. It is a place where you can go at any time.

Don't miss the "moments in-between."

Have you ever looked back at the end of a particularly busy day, with feelings of being stressed-out and fatigued, only to realize that the day was filled with minimal accomplishments? Part of the problem was that you missed the "moments in-between."

So often we spend much of our time rushing from one thing to the next just to end up waiting. Waiting for stop lights, waiting for appointments, and waiting for other people seem to be functions of modern life, but this has the potential of being the most valuable time of the day. Most of us spend it anxiously anticipating where we want to go or what we want to do, but it could be used for planning some other important part of our lives or, possibly more importantly, just meditating.

When life gets to be a bit too much, take time to pay attention to this particular moment. If you can, sit down and look for the good in this moment. Every moment of every day has something good about it. Let all other concerns slip away and for this brief period of time just appreciate being alive. Try to get in the habit of going through this simple thought process several times each day. If each moment is cherished for the good that it has to offer, then your outlook on life in general can only be positive.

HEALING MEDITATION

This special type of meditation has the potential of being one of the most powerful forms of healing. Emotional stress is a common part of chronic disease and cancer. This is true especially of conditions that cause pain. Regaining that sense of control is profoundly important in healing. Support from friends, family, and positive interactions with caregivers can increase control. Meditation, even in a basic form, is a very powerful tool for regaining a sense of control and decreasing the stress response associated with disease. Regular meditation provides an escape from pain, outside stressors, suffering, and discomfort. Having the ability to escape provides an increased sense of control over the situation. As an added benefit, adrenal function is improved and the immune system gets a boost.

The focus of healing meditation becomes the illness itself. This may be an injured part of the body or an area of pain. It may be a place in the body where cancer exists or it may be the body as a whole as in the case of a disease such as chronic fatigue or multiple sclerosis. Prayer can be included as a very important part of this meditation.

On a deeper level, healing meditation takes on a more spiritual quality. Beyond food, beyond exercise, beyond medications, beyond supplements, beyond herbal therapies and beyond simple relaxation, deep meditation is the key to healing. A deeper understanding of life and "self" must happen before true healing can occur. This understanding must reach a point where love of life goes beyond fear of losing it. Seek out an experienced individual to use as a guide when pursuing this level of meditation.

THE SPIRITUAL SIDE OF MEDITATION

Life is difficult and bad things happen. Meditation can be an avenue for escape from the difficulties of life, but it can be more. Anyone who meditates regularly will admit that there is something else; something that is beyond who we are. Describing it any further is difficult. The religions of the world have been trying to do so for all of time. It may be best to just accept that it is so and take comfort in the fact that we are never truly alone. Peace and comfort are always at hand, even in the most adverse of situations. Meditation, done without so much as a word or a thought, is the way to touch this concept most deeply.

A GOOD NIGHT'S SLEEP

The key to sleeping well at night is consistently having stress-controlled days. Regularly practicing methods to maintain low adrenaline levels during the day is very conducive to falling asleep normally at night and not waking in the middle of the night. Beyond stress reduction, here is some sound advice for restoring normal sleep cycles:

Avoid caffeine and other stimulants completely. Most beverages are available in caffeine-free versions. Look for hidden stimulants in supplements and foods. Be aware that many if not most medications disrupt stage 3 and 4 sleep. Avoid alcoholic beverages in the evening. Alcohol itself is a sedative, but its metabolites are stimulants. Expect to be wide-eyed and awake about 3 to 4 hours later.

Be very particular about bedtime routines. Try to set a pattern of going to bed and getting up at the same time each day. Respect normal day and night cycles as much as possible. If you work an odd shift, use darkening shades to completely darken the room where you sleep.

Avoid excessive light stimulation in the evening. Use low lights and turn off televisions and especially computer screens after 8 pm. This will help stimulate natural melatonin levels. Try reading before bedtime or practicing relaxation techniques.

Always sleep in a very dark room.

Avoid exercise after 8 pm except for relaxing yoga routines.

*Sleeping pills would seem like the simplest solution to insomnia, but there is absolutely **no substitute** for natural sleep. Sleep-inducing medications are* *often useful for transient insomnia, but are never ideal for long-term therapy. Taking sleeping pills will quickly prevent your body from returning to a natural rhythm of sleep. If you use sleeping pills chronically, be prepared to "pay the piper," as all sleep- inducing medications suppress natural sleep mechanisms of the body and tolerance develops. At some point you will have to stop taking the sleeping pills and it may not be easy.*

When searching for solutions to chronic insomnia, look for a healthcare practitioner who is skilled in evaluating and treating different forms of insomnia without using potent pharmaceuticals. Supplements are available that are not only safe but also effective, if combined with the proper lifestyle modifications.

SOMETIMES YOU HAVE TO ROW YOUR OWN BOAT

Life is hard. Life is hard, not for just a few but for each of us. The difficulties of life are different for each individual—we each have our own boat to row. Good or bad, our destiny shapes who we are. We must learn to accept our destiny and make the absolute best out of it. Lamenting what could have been and might have been only makes suffering worse.

Stress seems to always be pushing us. Often the push is uncomfortable, but the direction of the push is a matter of outlook. Those who are able to find a silver lining generally end up with a positive outcome. Following the push of stress to a positive end requires vision, acceptance, tolerance and sometimes humility.

Being caught up in the vicious pace of a rat-race lifestyle often causes suffering. Relaxation techniques and meditation are effective tools for dealing with emotional stress in the short term, but an overly stressful lifestyle needs a long-term solution. The first order of business in this regard is putting things into perspective. Often our life situation is not as bad as we perceive it to be. The second is recognizing that we have more control over our life situation than we often allow. Simple changes in the way we go about life can dramatically reduce daily stress.

Learn to accept your own pathway in life, even though it may be different from those around you.

THINGS THAT SEEM TO BE THREATENING, BUT ARE NOT

Anxiety is synonymous with fear—fear of the unknown, fear of things that seem beyond our abilities, fear of losing control; it all adds up. Be reassured that obstacles are rarely as big as they seem and things are rarely as bad as your mind makes them out to be.

Think of all the obstacles you have overcome in your life. You will overcome the ones before you just as well. Our abilities are always greater than we give ourselves credit for. Remind yourself of this every day.

STRESS CAUSED BY OTHER PEOPLE

Interacting with other people can certainly be a source of stress. When it comes to negative interactions with bosses and co-workers, make sure that your own fears, anxiety or arrogance are not contributing to the problem. In dealing with someone whose behavior you deem unacceptable, recognize that though your paths are presently intertwined, your destinies may be quite different. Things will inevitably change over time.

No matter how hard you try, you will never please everyone.

Responding negatively to negativism can only make a bad situation worse.

Make the best of the present and prepare for the future. If your present work situation is unacceptable, use it as a platform for learning about people in general and yourself and move toward change in the future. Use the techniques found in this chapter for dealing with stress to make the best of the situation until change can happen. Who knows, one day you might be running the company.

Stand up for what you believe in, but pick your battles well. Much stress and anxiety is created over trivial matters. Some things need to just roll off your shoulders. Before acting on a matter, ask yourself whether it is significant enough for the bother. Does action have the potential to cause more grief in the long run? If the matter is significant, look for positive avenues for resolution, such that everyone wins in the end.

Do not let others pull you down. Accept that you only have so much influence over those around you. Emotionally unstable individuals tend to drain energy from the people closest to them. In certain situations distance is required. It is also impossible for you to help someone else unless you are emotionally stable. When it comes to children, know that the greatest influence you have is by the example you set. If you have set a poor example, be willing to tolerate the consequences.

Stress is often caused by having to deal with illness in a loved one. Caring for someone who is very ill is draining, both physically and emotionally, especially if that person is in pain. That person may not be able to change his or her situation and may become increasingly dependent on you. Do whatever you can to help out, but remember to reserve some time and space for yourself. Get help from others whenever possible. You do not have to do it all yourself. Keeping up your strength is essential for helping someone else.

SELF-IMPOSED STRESS

Sometimes we voluntarily impose stress on ourselves. Stress is often required to "get ahead" and improve our standing in life, but the vicious cycle of working harder to gain more can become self-defeating. It is better to have a well-defined plan with specific and reasonable goals in mind.

The soccer mom (dad) syndrome. Many kids follow a schedule that would challenge the CEO of a major corporation. Many parents live vicariously and follow an equally demanding routine. Even "down time" is a scheduled event.

We are teaching our kids not only to be competitive, but also to be anxious and uptight. In the process, we are making life, in general, overly structured and uncomfortable.

Typically, when I counsel patients suffering from mental stress, I often find that an overly structured life is contributing to their misery. They are caught up in a vortex, and breaking free is nearly impossible. When I suggest a less structured lifestyle, meditation, or casual exercise, they quickly insist that they lack time.

Outside of normal sleep, unstructured time is the most health-friendly time of the day. Adrenaline decreases and contentment increases. Exercise is much more beneficial and enjoyable if not relegated to a time slot. Unstructured does not necessarily mean nonproductive. It just means not *having* to produce or to follow any particular time schedule. Any type of activity is more meaningful if not constrained by time limits and necessity.

Build space into your life for unstructured time. It can be used to accomplish a goal, such as better health, but sometimes it can best be used to accomplish nothing more than to take time to reflect on life.

DEALING WITH TRAUMATIC STRESS

If you have been through a harrowing experience, first you must stabilize your life by eliminating as many stress factors as possible and then rebuild slowly from there. Gather all resources at your disposal. Lean on others you can trust as much as you can without being an imposition. Get help with the kids. Take time off from work, if possible. Manage only absolute necessities and let everything else go.

Your daily goal should be to keep your adrenaline levels as low as possible. With time, the chemical imbalances in the brain that cause anxiety and depression will resolve. Moderate exercise is important, but activities should be pleasant and positive. Walking for 30 minutes is a simple but surprisingly effective antidepressant.

Avoid news media so that you can focus on recovery. The latest exploits of politicians and TV-stars are not your primary concerns. Read books and watch movies or television only if the topics are uplifting or positive. Above all, avoid associating with negative people; instead, seek out individuals with positive outlooks.

Fill your life with as much positive thought and feeling as possible.

LETTING GO OF STRESS

The feeling of letting go of all stress and all negative emotions is like none other. You may have felt it after walking away from a difficult exam (especially if you felt good about it) or maybe at the beginning of a vacation, as you distanced yourself from the regular responsibilities and work. It may have occurred after intense exercise, with the buildup of natural endorphins in your system. You may have also felt it just after the first beer on Saturday night (but less so with each additional bottle). Release from stress and anxiety can occur with a dose of Xanax or Valium, but in an artificial kind of way. The effects are transient and each subsequent dose provides less and less of a response.

Being able to feel this kind of release is a very important part of health. Unfortunately, having a feeling of total release does not happen spontaneously very often. All of the suggestions and exercises found in this chapter are designed to reduce stress, but sometimes you just have to let go. As a summary and a reminder, I will leave you with the following inspiration. Read it daily, if you like. If you follow it and believe in it, it will become a powerful force in your life.

I will look for the positive in every moment of every hour of every day, for negative emotions are a waste of precious time.

I will work to negotiate a better situation for myself in life, but at the same time I will not take advantage of others or cause others ill will.

I will set reasonable goals for myself and work every day to accomplish those goals, recognizing that some days will be better than others. I am only human.

I will let go of things that I can do nothing about, because I know that worrying about things beyond my control is very destructive.

I will look for the good in every individual, but I will not allow myself to be abused or taken advantage of.

I will let go of negative people in my life. I will either help them change or leave them behind.

I will let go of stress, for it can only do me harm.

Conclusion
and a new beginning...

Change is part of the mystery of life. About the time you decide that life is not worth living, change happens and everything falls into place. Looking backwards, you realize that the positive change that finally occurred would never have been possible without the pain that preceded it.

Controlling all of life's variables is impossible. We do, however, have control over many aspects of our lives, often more than we realize or take advantage of. Choices are as much a part of life as change. The choices we make when confronted with change will greatly influence our total life experience. Pursuing choices that positively influence our chances for good health influence our life experience more than any other factor.

YOU are the only one who can change your life.

Time's wasting.

Start making a plan now!

CREATING YOUR OWN ISLAND

It is possible to create your own "island" within the world in which you live. You may already have some ideas about how you would like yours to be. Creating an island within your own world is a matter of making choices—choices about the types of food you are willing to purchase, the amount of time you are willing to devote to work, the type of job you are willing to have, and how much personal time you set aside for your own health and well-being.

It is a material world and your island will require certain material things, but priorities are important. Things that you cannot do without—food, water, companionship, shelter and money—can be considered essentials. Your world should be structured such that these essentials are safe from most threats, but they also should be maintained at a level that does not cause stress. In other words, if you are working three jobs to afford a higher standard of living, then maybe it is time to reprioritize. Luxury items should only contribute to your life in a positive way, never in a stress-inducing manner.

THE CONCEPT OF WORK

Work (paid or unpaid) can help define who we are. There is something to be said for a job well done. Though it can define you, it also can consume you. Too many people struggle in jobs they do not enjoy to be able to afford things they do not really need. Find a job that you can enjoy. Job satisfaction can help to elevate your mood, reduce your stress and improve your health.

MATERIAL THINGS: PUTTING YOUR WANTS INTO PERSPECTIVE

There is nothing wrong with getting ahead in life, but always keep your priorities in order. The first priority for happiness is health, for without good health nothing else really matters. The second priority is happiness in love and relationships, for which devotion and self-sacrifice are required. Well behind the first two, a third priority includes material things. Such "wants" are often a source of misery instead of pleasure when not placed into proper perspective.

When an object of desire is sought for the positive experiences it may provide, the outcome is generally good.

When an object of desire is coveted just for the sake of having it, the repercussions are generally negative.

Ask yourself, does the object you desire have the potential to enrich your life?

An object of desire does not necessarily have to be material. You may desire a higher position in your employment for improved status and better pay; but is the increased stress worth it? Will it have a positive or an adverse effect on other aspects of your life?

Keep your financial concerns simple. If frugality has not been your practice, consolidate all of your debts into one loan and make a pledge to never to become over-extended again.

Much of life's misery arises from the never ending pursuit of unrealistic goals and perpetual dissatisfaction with the present moment.

In the long run, strive for realistic goals and be willing to accept some compromises.

The game is always changing. Learn to accept change and to change with change.

Contentment means not wanting for anything.
True happiness is wanting everything you have.

IT'S A MATTER OF TIME

We each have twenty-four hours in every day, but rarely does it seem to be enough. At least eight hours should be allotted for sleep and many of us are obligated to eight hours of work. If work consumes more than eight hours on most days, then it may be time to reevaluate your concept of work. After work and sleep, about eight hours are left for all of life's other activities.

Of those eight hours, a certain amount of time will be necessary for preparing food, paying bills, caring for spouses/children and other life concerns, but some time should be left unstructured. Unstructured time is not the same as wasted time. Unstructured time is your personal time for activities such as exercise, meditation, reading, writing or other hobbies. Unlike sitting in front of a television, these activities are productive and contribute to your health in a positive way.

Unstructured time is the most important time of the day. It is your time to gain on life instead being beaten down by it. Health and happiness are often directly related to the amount of unstructured time allowed each day. When planning priorities, unstructured time should always have a place near the top.

LIVING WITHIN YOUR GENES

For health, the limiting factor is often our genes. Our genetic makeup defines our tolerance to foods, our threshold for disease, how we deal with stress and, to a certain extent, our outlook on life. Going against your genes will only get you into trouble. Listen to your body and do what feels right. If certain foods make you feel bad (even if they taste good), it's time to let them go. The same goes for many other aspects of life. Pursue activities that make you feel alive. Some people are born to dance and others express themselves through painting. Find your own niche, and go where life leads you.

IT'S A SMALL WORLD AFTER ALL

Part of creating your own island is making your world smaller and simpler. So much of what comes through the news media is sensationalized and does not have a direct impact on your life. Filter your news intake if it tends to cause anxiety. Consider taking periodic vacations from news media. You will be surprised at how little you will miss. If you want to know more about the world, read a travel novel or *National Geographic* for a less sensational approach. Reading about history is reassuring; you will note that humans have not changed very much in all of recorded time and the world is probably no worse off than it has ever been.

Making your world smaller extends to your relationships with other people. To some extent, you can choose who you allow on your island. Look for meaningful relationships that pick you up instead of dragging you down.

Another part of creating your own island is having a positive outlook on life. Try to see the good in other people and overlook the bad. Remember that you are only human and others around you are the same. Tolerance is, indeed, one of the most important virtues we can achieve as human beings. Smile more often, even if you don't feel like it. Also remember that every day is not going to be a "great" day, but tomorrow could be the best yet. It is amazing how quickly life can turn around with the right outlook.

THE FOUR YEAR PLAN

"Creating your own island" is not something that happens overnight. I think anyone who has been caught up in a rat-race lifestyle has been tempted to just walk away, but life is never quite so simple. Loyalty to a hard-won career, even if it is a major source of stress, is hard to give up. A spouse's career, kids in school, and dependence on those material things that seem so important tend to get in the way. A real change in lifestyle takes time, effort, and, most importantly, a plan.

Think ahead as to what kinds of changes you would like to make in your life over the next four years. Four years seems to be a realistic time interval for most people to make real change. Take stock of what you really need to be content. Are you at the point in life where you could consider some type of retirement or choose a less stressful job that gives greater contentment? Down-sizing your home and living expenses may be a part of the plan. Taking better care of your health by taking more time for relaxation, exercise, and cooking better food should be an essential part of the change. As you make a plan, decide what stage you would like to be at in one year, two years, three years, and ultimately in four years. The stress of change may be part of the picture, but ultimately you will be more relaxed, content, and healthier.

OVERCOMING AND RECOVERING FROM ILLNESS

Sometimes a change in lifestyle is forced by a significant illness. The above considerations apply, but must be followed more intensively. While trying to regain health after a serious illness, you should be especially conscientious about how you live life. All potential stress factors that may contribute to maintaining a state of chronic disease must be reduced or eliminated. After healing has occurred and health is recovered, a more normal life can be resumed and more stress can be tolerated.

The concept of threshold is very important in understanding chronic disease. Chronic disease does not happen suddenly; rather, it occurs insidiously. The forces that cause disease are present and causing subtle but cumulative damage long before symptoms arise. A state that could be defined as "pre-disease" occurs, with the patient asymptomatic and unaware, until a certain threshold defined by our genes is crossed and suddenly a cascade of symptoms ensues. Symptoms gradually increase and coalesce into a well-defined disease process.

The time between onset of symptoms and absolute diagnosis is often quite protracted; by then, more than one diagnosis may be present. Any point along this continuum is the time to act, but the earlier the better, of course. Even if a diagnosis has been made, most chronic disease processes can be reversed if the pressures are released. Recognize that chronic disease does have well-defined causes, but the causes are multi-factorial. Stress factors must be reduced to below threshold levels and kept there long enough for healing to occur. Basic guidelines for optimizing your healing potential include the following:

If you suffer from a chronic disease, take control of your own situation. Spend more effort searching for reversible causes that have contributed to your disease than worrying about your diagnosis. Restoring balance is the key to restoring health.

If your condition has not yet been firmly diagnosed, you may still benefit from some of these suggestions.

The recommendations for healthy food and eating are extremely important. Avoid almost all meat and processed food while recovering from an illness. Meat, dairy, processed corn, sugar and wheat products are the primary inflammatory foods, and these should be avoided completely during recovery. Especially avoid any processed sugars and starches. A healthy daily allotment of vegetables and fruit are essential. Fresh, organic food is essential. Avoid foods containing any types of chemical additives. The healthiest way of cooking food is steaming. Avoid grilled or fried foods and overly-cooked food.

To gain extra nutrients, consider juicing organic fruits and vegetables daily.

Drink plenty of clean, pure water.

Nutritional supplements can be beneficial for the transition toward better health. Pursue the advice of a qualified healthcare provider in choosing an appropriate regimen of supplements. (See Appendix C as well as the last page of the references.)

Take medications as directed by your healthcare provider, but be aware that sometimes side effects from medications can impede healing. Many medications suppress the immune system and/or have the potential to induce vitamin and mineral deficiencies. As you become healthier you may be able to reduce the dosages of some medications. Try to avoid becoming over-medicated.

Have your thyroid and other basic labs checked. Abnormal thyroid function often accompanies chronic disease. (See Appendix B for basic recommended labs.)

Manage insulin resistance and diabetes aggressively. High insulin levels adversely affect other hormone systems of the body, and baseline (fasting) blood glucose levels in the 95-110 range (even though considered normal) impede healing functions of the body. Normalize insulin and blood glucose levels by whatever means necessary.

Become acutely "toxin aware" and avoid exposure to toxins as much as possible. Hidden or unrecognized toxins can be an underlying factor in any chronic disease. An appropriately designed detoxification protocol can often improve your energy and augment healing. Review the recommendations in Chapter 11.

Try far-infrared sauna treatments. Some experts consider this to be an essential part of detoxification. Define a treatment protocol with your healthcare provider.

Alcohol and caffeine should be avoided until you are well.

Regular exercise is essential for overcoming chronic disease. Even if the extent of your ability is walking around the living room three times, do it regularly until you can do more. Work up gradually. Though exercise is beneficial, it is important not to over-tax the body. The regular practice of yoga can be very beneficial for a healing body.

Make your world as "small" and stress-free as possible. You may have to rely on other people you can trust and cut back on your day-to-day needs and living expenses. You will likely discover a "stress threshold" that precipitates symptoms. Try to maintain stress below the threshold.

Remember, adrenaline is the enemy when trying to recover from chronic disease. Anything you can do to consistently lessen your adrenaline levels is beneficial. As your health improves, you will be able to tolerate more stress and enjoy a little more freedom.

Avoid becoming upset about things that you have no control over. This is extremely counter-productive because it detracts from your focus on healing and recovering.

Meditation is the most powerful healing tool I know of. Become familiar with techniques of meditation or self-relaxation and practice them as often as you can.

Pray regularly.

Rest often during the day and make sure you are getting plenty of sleep. Seven or more hours every night is optimal. Natural and pharmaceutical sleep aids may be indicated, but use them cautiously and wisely. Avoid medications known to suppress the immune system or cause habituation.

Establish a relationship with a healthcare provider who is willing to listen and offer guidance, without dictating therapy. A thorough evaluation is sometimes indicated to uncover hidden threats that may respond to targeted therapy.

The start of each day provides a new opportunity to renew your health. Take advantage of it. Concentrate all of your efforts on that goal.

Look for the positive moments in every day and try to generate as much of a positive outlook on life as you can. Smile, even when you do not feel like it. I cannot tell you how important this is in overall healing.

Absolutely anything can be improved with motivation and a positive attitude. You can become well again!

BRIEF EPILOG

With persistent effort my health rebounded, but I recognize the need for continual vigilance—good health is not something to be taken for granted. Stress and genetics probably played a significant role in the insomnia and fatigue I experienced throughout my forties, but a tick bite and a test indicating possible exposure to the bacterium that causes Lyme disease may have also been a factor. I may never know for sure—at present I remain happily free of a diagnosis.

I am content with my life and my health for right now, but I recognize the need for periodic change. My next four year plan may be to look for that perfect island. I am sure it actually exists somewhere, possibly in the Caribbean or the Greek Isles. I probably wouldn't stay, but it sure would be a pleasure to go and look around!

Appendix A

SCREENING LABS

LEVEL 1 BASIC ASSESSMENT

- **Complete blood count**   Count of red blood cells and inflammatory cells. Measures hemoglobin for detection of anemia.

- **Metabolic panel**   Measures basic blood chemistry, liver function and kidney function. Includes fasting blood glucose.

- **Lipid profile**   Measures triglycerides and cholesterol. Shows total cholesterol as well as the breakdown by particle types HDL ("good") and LDL ("bad") cholesterol.   Satisfactory screening for individuals under age fifty with no risk factors. Includes C-reactive protein as a screen for inflammatory risks associated with atherosclerosis.

- **Thyroid screen**   Thyroid stimulating hormone (TSH) is used for basic screening purposes in individuals with a positive family history or in asymptomatic women over age fifty.

LEVEL 2 OVER AGE 50 OR WITH RISK FACTORS

- **Advanced atherosclerosis screening**   For all individuals over age fifty and individuals under fifty with any risk factors.

Includes complete lipoprotein particle profile (determines particle size) and C-reactive protein.

- **Hemoglobin A1c and fasting insulin** Screening for insulin resistance and early onset diabetes. Because "protein-sticking" is such an significant factor in aging, hemoglobin A1c is an important test for monitoring rate of aging.

- **Essential fatty acids (AA/EPA ratio)** The ratio of omega-6 to omega-3 fatty acids can be measured by special testing. The ideal ratio for a low inflammatory response is 4:1. This ratio is commonly found in the traditional Japanese population who demonstrate the greatest longevity and lowest risk of cardiovascular disease in the world. The ratio of most average Americans is closer to 11:1. Inflammatory conditions and neurologic disorders are common at 20:1. Determining the body saturation of omega-3s may prove to be one of the most sensitive indicators for predicting stroke and heart attack.

- **Micronutrient profile** Testing for deficiencies in specific vitamins and minerals. Assays for vitamin D, vitamin B-12, and minerals (including calcium and magnesium) can be ordered through standard labs. Types of testing can be defined by a qualified healthcare provider.

- **Complete hormone profile** DHEAS, testosterone, estradiol, estrone, and progesterone. Blood testing is most accurate, but only offers a snapshot in time. Salivary hormone testing offers a broader analysis, but is much less accurate. Salivary testing is best for guiding hormone replacement therapy. (Indicated if fatigue or hormonal dysfunction are present.) DHEAS is an adrenal hormone that declines with age. Decline is considered a marker for premature aging.

- **Complete thyroid testing** Includes thyroid stimulating hormone (TSH) and free (active) thyroid hormones T-3 and T-4. Thyroid antibody testing may be ordered in certain situations when symptoms consistent with hypothyroidism persist despite normal hormone levels. Thyroid antibody testing includes thyroid peroxidase (TPO) and anti-thyroglobulin antibody. (Indicated if fatigue is present.)

- **Risk of thrombosis** A small percentage of people are "hyper-coagulators" and are at risk for thrombotic events (blood clots). Screening labs for genetic susceptibility include Leiden factor V, homocysteine, protein C deficiency, protein S deficiency and antithrombin. These tests should be considered in anyone with a family history of thrombotic events, especially if estrogen products are being considered.

LEVEL 3 HISTORY OF CHRONIC DISEASE

- **3-hour glucose tolerance test with insulin levels** Indicated when insulin resistance or diabetes is suspected.

- **Food sensitivity testing** Food sensitivities are often an underlying factor in chronic disease. This can be a beneficial adjunct to an elimination diet. Different panels are available for food and airborne allergies.

- **24-hour cortisol levels** Salivary hormones are tested at four different times during the day. (Cortisol concentrations are much higher than other adrenal and reproductive hormones, so salivary levels are valid for testing.) (Quest labs) Indicated primarily in cases of chronic fatigue that are refractory to therapy.

- **TB skin test** Recommended if lung disease or possible exposure has been present.

- **Heavy metal testing** Heavy metal toxicity can be a factor in chronic disease. Total RBC concentration can be used as a screen for acute exposure, but if chronic toxicity is suspected, the best measurement involves 24-hour urine collection after stimulation with DMSA. (Hair samples are not always accurate because detergents in daily shampoo can add to or wash out toxic substances.)

- **Lyme disease testing** Indicated when chronic fatigue and arthritis are present.

- **Rheumatoid factor / ANA titer**   Indicated when arthritis or suspicions of autoimmune disease are present.

- **HIV, Syphilis and Hepatitis**   If sexually transmitted disease suspected.

Specific recommendations for laboratory evaluation should be defined by a qualified healthcare provider.

Appendix B:

EVERYDAY SUPPLEMENTS FOR OPTIMAL HEALTH

Natural supplements are not a substitute for a healthful diet, but they can complement wise food choices. Important disease-reducing chemical compounds found in foods or herbs can be concentrated in supplement form for maximal benefit. Unlike foods, which have a primary purpose of providing calories, natural supplements provide intense doses of vital nutrients to inhibit processes of disease.

The concept of consuming concentrated plant substances to provide health restoring or medicinal value is not a new one. Herbal medicine has been around a long time. Records of the medicinal use of herbs date back at least 5000 years and surely herbs were used even before recorded history. You can imagine our primitive man going about his day gathering food. He learned which plants would harm him and which plants would help him. Some plants likely would have been eaten for the sole purpose of reducing symptoms or simply to make him feel well.

The key to using natural supplements appropriately is letting Mother Nature be the ultimate guide. Sometimes this requires as much common sense as science. The best supplements are in their purest, most natural forms, free of contaminants and highly standardized, such that benefit is reliably predictable. Natural supplements should be presented to the body in a form that is as readily absorbable and is as easily assimilated as any food.

Nutritional supplements come in many forms, with tablets, capsules, liquids and tinctures being the most common. Most often the form is a matter of personal preference, but sometimes it can make a difference. Probiotics and some enzyme preparations need to be enteric coated for protection against stomach acid. Others, such as melatonin and vitamin B-12 are best delivered under the tongue as sublingual preparations. Tinctures are the most rapidly absorbed herbal supplements but are often quite bitter and are therefore not preferred by most people.

Liquid supplements with ingredients dissolved in fruit juice or flavored liquid are very popular but are generally not the best option. Liquid supplements tend to be very high in sugar and are limited to ingredients that taste good. This is a very significant limitation, because many very important ingredients are quite bitter. It seems that for most supplements, capsules are the preferred vehicle for delivery. Capsules go down better than tablets and can be designed to deliver a wide range of products. A viscous liquid such as soy milk or almond milk (with a taste of chocolate syrup) makes taking capsules effortless.

Each of the supplements listed below can be found at www.vitalplan.com.

PREVENT

Essential Fatty Acids (EFA)

The scientific evidence in favor of supplementing with essential fatty acids is hard to ignore. Essential fatty acids (EFAs) are important for decreasing inflammation in the body, supporting optimal cell membrane function and improving brain function. The incidences of virtually all chronic diseases and some cancers are significantly reduced by having the proper concentration of omega-3 fatty acids. Though all types of essential fatty acid supplements reduce inflammation, marine sources are especially important for inhibiting the processes that cause damaging arterial plaques associated with heart attacks and stroke. In fact, a daily dose of quality fish or krill oil may be as effective at reducing heart disease as any drug on the market. Vegetable sources of essential fatty acids are better for reducing general inflammation, such as that associated with arthritis.

Natural sources of essential fatty acids include oily fish, Antarctic krill, flaxseed oil, borage oil, walnuts and a healthful diet in general. Of all the sources, krill, a minute shrimp harvested in Antarctica, has moved to the top of the list. The omega-3 fats found in krill are more stable than those found in fish and also are more readily absorbed. This form, called a phospholipid, offers unique properties that are readily utilized by the body. This translates into smaller doses with no fishy taste—ever. In addition, krill oil contains a potent natural antioxidant, called astaxanthin, which lowers risk of cardiovascular disease and inflammatory conditions such as arthritis. Krill is a very sustainable resource; maximal harvest is predicted to only affect 1% of the total Antarctic supply.

Fish oil is still the most common EFA supplement choice, and it is a good choice, as long as the standard of quality is kept high. Freshness is the key. Oxidation (spoilage) can occur during the manufacturing process or if the product sits on the shelf too long. A high-quality supplement should not have a "fishy" smell or taste. EFA supplements should be taken as a single ingredient supplement, because spoilage is more likely if they are combined with other ingredients. Refrigeration is essential for maintaining shelf-life of fish oil supplements, both before and after purchase.

Antioxidants

When healthy people who follow a healthful diet undergo nutritional assessment, the one area in which they often fall short is adequate antioxidant protection. Though daily consumption of adequate amounts of fruit and vegetables is essential, natural supplements provide concentrated antioxidant support without adding sugar. Though there are many natural substances known to provide antioxidant protection, the following list details some of the most well studied. These ingredients can be collectively found in the supplement **Prevention Plus™**.

> **Resveratrol**, found in grapes and in a plant called Japanese knotweed, offers potent antioxidant protection for the cardiovascular system. It also is known to have anti-microbial properties and immune-enhancing properties.

> **French maritime pine bark**, full of potent substances offering anti-inflammatory and anti-oxidant properties. Studies have shown positive benefit for reducing blood pressure, improving athletic performance, and improving circulation (especially diabetics). There is some evidence to support cholesterol reduction and improvement in blood sugar control in diabetics.

Milk thistle (Silymarin), well-known to offer liver protection, is vital for reducing risk of disease. Milk thistle increases bile flow, protects liver cells from the detoxification process and has actually been shown to induce regeneration of liver cells.

Lutein, the yellow pigment found in vegetables, when combined with its isomer, ***zeaxanthin***, protects both the retina of the eyes and skin from the damaging effects of the sun. The colorful pigments found in ***bilberries*** or ***blueberries*** offer similar protection.

Astaxanthin, the chemical compound responsible for the pink color found in salmon and shrimp, may be the most potent antioxidant known. Not only does it offer protection to skin and eyes, but it also reduces tissue inflammation and reduces cancer and cardiovascular disease risk.

Quercetin, known for antihistamine properties and blood vessel health is important for protecting cardiovascular function. ***Rutin*** is a similar substance offering the same benefit.

Pomegranate, noted for antioxidant properties and positive effects on blood pressure and

Acai berry, known for reducing cholesterol.

Lycopene, the red pigment found in tomato sauce and catsup, has been found to inhibit breast cancer cells and prostate cancer cells.

The Basic Multivitamin

The question of whether to take a multivitamin is quite controversial. On one hand, information suggests that our requirements for vitamins and minerals go up as we age, even in people who follow healthy diets. On the other hand, clinical studies have consistently shown no benefit and even possible detriment from taking a multivitamin. It must be taken into account, however, that these studies were done with synthetically-derived vitamins.

A perfect diet is the logical answer, but even individuals who strive for this goal admit that eating the perfect diet every day is challenging. A multivitamin could fill dietary voids, but special care must be taken in choosing the correct formulation. The basic "once a day," composed of synthetic vitamins "dumped" into the system at one time, is clearly not the best option. Common sense alone would suggest that consumption of synthetically-derived vitamins and inorganic forms of minerals could do more harm than good.

The simple answer is moderation and following nature's lead. Healthy food should be the primary source of essential vitamins and minerals, with supplements providing the very minimums to ensure against deficiencies. Vitamins should be presented to the body in natural activated forms that are readily absorbed and assimilated. The same goes for minerals, which should be present in natural organic forms, not as the inorganic forms found in most multivitamin supplements.

Key indicators of a good multivitamin include the following:
- Natural carotenes instead of high levels of vitamin A, which can build up in fatty tissues and be toxic
- Having the full spectrum of natural forms of vitamin E instead of d-alpha tocopherol alone
- Having natural folates instead of folic acid. Because folic acid is a cell growth initiator, daily doses of 400-800 mcg have been associated with increased cancer risk. Outside of pregnancy there is no indication for folate doses >400 mcg.
- The other B vitamins should be represented in full spectrum.
- Iodine is a desirable ingredient, but copper is generally not.
- No added iron. Most people consuming a healthy diet get enough iron from food and supplementation is only indicated when anemia is present.
- All minerals should be in natural, organic form instead of inorganic—you don't want rocks in your multivitamin.

Prevention Plus™ provides a balanced complement of essential vitamins found in activated form and organic minerals.

OPTIMIZE

Bone and Joint Health

Expert opinion is shifting away from calcium supplements toward obtaining calcium primarily from dietary sources. Use of the most common types of calcium supplements have only marginally decreased fracture risk and have been associated with "hardening of arteries." Calcium is best obtained from sources such as leafy greens, figs and almonds. An alkalinizing diet, rich in vegetables, is essential for maintaining calcium within bones. Supplements should provide nutrients in ways that diet alone cannot. For the skeletal system, **Bone & Collagen Complex** is just that sort of supplement. Bone & Collagen Complex not only provides an important foundation for dietary calcium, but also provides essential nutrients for maintaining healthy joints, ligaments and bone structure support. Beyond Bone & Collagen Complex, have your vitamin D levels checked to be assured of proper vitamin D supplementation.

Staying active is probably one of the most important things you can do to maintain healthy bones and resist aging, but joint problems and arthritis can be an impediment to regular exercise, especially after age 50. **Joint Care** contains potent anti-inflammatory ingredients designed to reduce joint inflammation and protect joint function. As a bonus, two of the ingredients, turmeric and boswellia, may reduce cancer risk and dementia risk. Joint Care also contains glucosamine, important for maintaining healthy cartilage. When combined, **Joint Care** and **Bone & Collagen Complex** offer unprecedented coverage for the entire skeletal system.

Stress Management

For most of us, everyday emotional stress is a contributing factor to disease and aging. Moderating the effects of stress through daily mindfulness and practice of breathing and focus exercises reduce this risk factor, but certain supplements are also beneficial. **HPA Balance™**, a combination product containing patented forms of several thoughtfully chosen herbal ingredients, normalizes the stress response and balances hormonal and immune functions that have been disturbed by stress. Clinically this product is extremely effective and does not carry the safety concerns and habituation issues common with drug therapies.

Probiotics

Recognized as "old friends," regular oral inoculations of favorable bacteria are not only important for normal gastrointestinal function, but also for balancing and restoring normal immune function—important for everyday health, but essential for reducing chronic allergies and recovering from any type of intestinal dysfunction. Consumption of fermented foods providing friendly bacteria is an everyday affair in many parts of the world, but not in the U. S. With the exception of yogurt, fermented foods are rarely consumed by most Americans, and even yogurt is not a daily item for most people.

Accumulating evidence suggests that daily use of a probiotic supplement provides benefits similar to those gained by regularly consuming fermented foods. It potentially could be even more beneficial because inoculations are more regular and dosage and types of bacteria are controlled. Probiotics are now being recognized for therapeutic value in treating a wide range of medical problems. Consult **www.vitalplan.com** for further advice on selecting an everyday probiotic supplement.

Immune Modulators

A diverse group of immune-modulating substances known as beta-glucans are another type of "old friend" that help "reset" the immune system. Beta-glucans are found in fungal species such as mushrooms and certain types of yeast. All edible mushrooms contain some of these important substances, but the types of beta-glucans found in maitake, reishi and shitake mushrooms are becoming well known for reducing risks of autoimmune disease and cancer. Beyond regular consumption, supplements may be a way to gain the important health benefits offered by these substances.

Mitochondrial Support

Mitochondria, the microscopic football-shaped structures present in all living cells, provide energy necessary for all cellular functions. Generation of free radicals is an obligatory by-product of the energy production process. Free radicals have propensity to damage all structures within the cell, including cell membranes, proteins, and very importantly, DNA. No structures, however, take more of the brunt of the damage than the mitochondria themselves. A gradual decline in energy secondary to the wane in mitochondria is one of the important processes of aging.

Limiting free-radical damage is essential for life. Cells are armed with protective antioxidants, but the ability to generate these important these complex compounds declines with age and chronic disease. *Glutathione* is the primary antioxidant that protects cellular function. Natural sources of glutathione include asparagus, spinach, avocados, squash, garlic and melons. Antioxidant protection can be augmented by glutathione supplements, which also provide detoxification support and anti-viral properties. Glutathione that has been oxidized by free radicals can be "recharged" by *alpha-lipoic acid* and *N-acetyl cysteine (NAC)*. Superoxide dismutase, another important antioxidant found inside cells, is specific for dispatching the most damaging types of free radicals. It can also be found in supplement form.

CoEnzyme Q-10 and *l-carnitine* are key players in cellular energy production. Though cells have the ability to manufacture these substances, some of this ability is lost with aging and chronic disease. Supplementation may be beneficial for increasing energy in the body and for generating energy within the heart. Co-enzyme Q-10 supplements are especially important for individuals taking cholesterol-lowering medications (statins), because these medications lower CoQ-10 levels.

Glucose-modulating Supplements

Half of Americans over forty are on the way to becoming insulin resistant and many already have Type II diabetes. Dietary modifications are definitely in order, but in many cases damage has already been done. Certain natural supplements are able to enhance the body's ability to manage blood glucose levels. They also help normalize insulin levels and at the same, reduce carbohydrate cravings. Anyone with fasting blood glucose consistently over 100 should consider taking this type of supplement with every meal.

Many non-toxic substances found in nature positively affect glucose metabolism. Ingredients including *chromium, gymnema, fenugreek, bitter melon, cinnamon, vanadium, banaba*, and *alpha lipoic acid* have been to offer clinical benefit. Blood glucose should be monitored and additional medical therapy should be considered if fasting blood glucose is over 130 or if other indications of diabetes are present.

Mental Acuity and Cognition

There are actually many natural substances that slow mental decline and enhance cognitive function, but an herbal substance called bacopa is one that stands out as being safe for everyday use. Traditionally used in ayurvedic medicine (traditional medicine of India) for moderation of anxiety and insomnia, *bacopa* has now been recognized by modern science to support cognitive function and enhance memory. Independent clinical studies using *bacopa* have shown improved attention and memory in elderly patients and significant improvement and learning ability and memory in children.

These guidelines are very general. Individual needs may vary according to diet and health status. Consult a healthcare provider with knowledge in wellness-based medicine for choosing the best regimen of everyday supplements.

www.vitalplan.com The source for premium quality, natural supplements

An opinion on aspirin

A daily dose of enteric-coated aspirin, 81mg is recommended by many providers. Aspirin reduces inflammation and inhibits platelet aggregation (decreases clotting). There is good evidence that aspirin reduces risks of stroke caused by blood clots, heart attacks and colon cancer. Aspirin has, however, been associated with increased incidence of hemorrhagic stroke (stroke caused by rupture of blood vessels in the brain.) This is not surprising, because aspirin does nothing to strengthen the integrity of blood vessels; in fact, it may do the opposite.

Virtually all the daily supplements, with essential fatty acids leading the way, have blood-thinning properties. Unlike aspirin, essential fatty acids and the anti-inflammatory supplements actually improve the integrity of the vascular system. The supplements recommended would be expected to provide all of the benefits of aspirin (and more), without the risk.

Appendix C

MORE SIMPLE COOKING

QUICK SUPPERS

Healthy shrimp and grits (with quinoa instead of grits)

Try this version and you will never be satisfied with anything else. Shrimp are high in protein, calcium, vitamin B-12, and selenium, but very low in food energy. Shrimp are high in cholesterol, but tend to raise favorable HDL cholesterol more than LDL cholesterol. Because they are low in fat overall and high in omega-3 fatty acids, consumption of shrimp actually lowers the risk of atherosclerosis.

Shrimp, ½ to 1 lb. (depending on the number of people)

Onions, chopped

Red bell peppers, chopped

Celery, chopped

Garlic, minced

Hummus, a couple of large spoonfuls

Low-fat sour cream or yogurt, a couple of large spoonfuls

Old Bay (or similar) seasoning, a good shake

Hot red chili paste, ½ teaspoon

Salt to taste

Quinoa, several cups, precooked (1 cup quinoa, 2 cups water, salt; cook for 15 minutes)

Sauté shrimp, onions, pepper, celery and seasonings in olive oil with garlic and seasonings. Add in the hummus and sour cream. Stir in the quinoa and serve. A baked butternut squash goes well with this dish.

Beef, barley, and cabbage rolls

Barley is an underutilized grain. It works well when included in many varieties of dishes and can also be prepared and eaten as a hot breakfast cereal, similar to oatmeal. Barley is very good for the digestive tract, lowers cholesterol, aids in the removal of toxins from the body, and slows the absorption of glucose for 10-12 hours after it is consumed!

  Small free-range steak, sliced into small cubes
  ½ onion, chopped
  1-2 cups cooked hulled barley
  Several large steamed cabbage leaves
  ½ can pizza or tomato sauce

Barley cooks like rice. Add 1 cup hulled barley to 2 cups of water. Heat the water to boiling and then reduce to simmer. Cover and cook for about 40 minutes. Cook a double batch to use in other dishes or for breakfast.

While the cabbage leaves are being steamed, sauté the steak and onion in olive oil until brown. Add in the barley and sauce. Scoop the mixture into the cabbage leaves, roll, and place back into the same pan. Cover and simmer on low for a few minutes. This should be enough to serve 3-4 people.

Quick and Easy Turkey Dinner

  2 boneless turkey breasts (free range)
  4 large sweet potatoes
  Several stalks of broccoli

Grill or bake the turkey breast for about 30 minutes (medium-low on the grill, 350 degrees in the oven). A good marinade is olive oil, fresh lemon, and allspice-based seasoning. (Save one of the breasts for the wild rice and turkey casserole recipe found in the casserole section.)

Peel the sweet potatoes and slice into smaller pieces. Place in a pot, cover with water, and boil until tender. Remove from boiling water and drain. Mash with a large fork. Mix in 1 to 2 tbsp. margarine and 1 to 2 tbsp. brown sugar. Transfer to a baking dish and smooth out. Bake at 350 for about 20 to30 minutes.

Steam the broccoli and sprinkle with your choice of cheese.

Spinach and sausage
   Fresh (or frozen) spinach or Swiss chard
   Soy sausage (or regular, if you insist)
   Chopped onions
   Chopped mushrooms
   One or two eggs
   Soy sauce
   Cooked brown rice (or quinoa)

Sauté the onions, mushrooms and sausage in oil of your choice on low heat. Add the spinach (or chard). When the spinach is wilted, crack the eggs and stir them in until cooked. Season with soy sauce and serve over brown rice.

Tempeh sauté
Tempeh is a very healthy source of protein made from cultured soybeans. Properly prepared, tempeh is quite tasty. Tempeh keeps well in the refrigerator and is quick and easy to prepare.
   One package tempeh
   Sliced brown button mushrooms (any mushrooms can be used)
   Grated garlic
   Grated ginger
   Soy sauce
   Olive oil

Sauté all ingredients together over low to heat, covered part of the time, until the mushrooms are tender.
Serve with steamed greens.

Black rice, black beans

Black rice sounds exotic enough that I had to try it. After minimal searching, I found it at a local grocery on the rice and pasta aisle. Supposedly this heirloom rice was once reserved for the emperors of China.

 2 cups black rice—cooked
 1 can black beans
 1 stalk celery—sliced
 1/3 onion—chopped
 Handful of raisins for sweetness
 ½ - 1 teaspoon cumin
 Splash of white wine
 Slivered almonds or cashews
 ¼ c. shredded cheese—any white cheese (Romano, fresh parmesan, or Monterey jack)
 Sea salt to taste
 Olive oil

Cook the black rice as per directions on the package in a 1½ - 2 quart pot. When cooked, the rice actually has a deep purple color and gives off a wonderful nutty aroma. Sauté celery and onions in olive oil. Add in cumin, salt, black beans, and wine; simmer covered for several minutes. Stir this sautéed mixture in with the rice. Add in the raisins, almonds, and cheese. Serve with a steamed vegetable and a glass of white wine—a truly sophisticated meal that takes no time at all to prepare.

Salmon and Greens

 1/2 to 1 lb. fresh salmon
 Bottled red pepper vinaigrette dressing (any brand)
 1-2 bunches (more than you think) of fresh greens (collards, kale, Swiss chard)
 1-2 cups sliced mushrooms
 ½ cup chopped green onions
 1-2 tsp. minced garlic
 1-2 tsp. rice vinegar
 2-3 tbs. olive oil

1-2 tsp. sesame oil
salt, paprika, and cayenne pepper to taste
sliced fresh plums
Yellow squash, chopped
Sweet onions, chopped

Steam the salmon (coated with the roasted red pepper dressing) for 5-10 minutes. Grilling also works well.

Chop the greens. This is done by laying the leaves on a chopping board and cutting cross sections about 1-inch thick with a large knife. In a deep pan, sauté the greens in olive and sesame oil with the mushrooms, onions and garlic. Throw them in, all at once, until the pan is packed to overflowing, and cover. Stir every minute or two until the greens are steamed down and soft.

Steam the squash and onions for about 6 to 8 minutes and top with your choice of cheese.

Serve the salmon and greens side-by-side, with the plums as a garnish. The squash is a side dish.

Cilantro Shrimp
1 lb. shrimp
1 thinly sliced orange bell pepper
1 thinly sliced tomato
1 thinly sliced zucchini squash
2 tbs. (about) fresh minced cilantro
1-2 tsp (about) minced garlic
Paprika to taste
Cayenne pepper to taste
Salt to taste
1-2 tbs. olive oil
½-1 cup grated parmesan or Monterey Jack cheese
Splash of soy milk
Whole grain pasta (optional)

Sauté shrimp, peppers, tomato, zucchini, cilantro, garlic, spices in olive oil. Add cheese and soy milk. Mix until cheese is completely melted. Serve with baked winter squash and hot tea to drink.

Back porch summer supper

Fresh bluefish with salt, pepper and olive oil, grilled on low for about 15 minutes.

Steamed corn on the cob with just a pat of butter.

Sliced tomato grown in the backyard.

Fresh green salad with walnuts, blueberries, and blackberry vinaigrette dressing.

This dish takes less than 30 minutes to prepare and 5 minutes to wash dishes.

Pesto chicken
> Boneless chicken breasts – one per person
> Sweet onion, sliced into round sections
> Pesto: (Grind together in food processor)
>>   1/2 cup fresh pine nuts
>>   1/4 c. olive oil
>>   1/2 c. freshly grated parmesan cheese
>>   1-3 tablespoons minced garlic
>>   Fresh minced or dried herbs (basil and oregano work well)
>>   Squeeze of fresh lemon

Pesto is most commonly found combined with pasta, but it has many uses in cooking. There are many different types and combinations of pesto, but a common ingredient is often pine nuts. Do not shy away from pine nuts when you see the fat content, as they are favorable fats. Pine nuts are rich in anti-oxidants and have a reputation as a natural appetite suppressant. Once you make your pesto, freeze the extra (in an ice-cube tray) for use at another time.

For this dish place the chicken breasts on top of the sliced onions in a glass baking dish. Cover the chicken with the remaining onion slices. Bake at 350 degrees for 30 minutes. Remove the top layer of onions. Spread pesto over the top of the chicken and bake for another 20 minutes.

Baked red potatoes or sweet potatoes and steamed sweet peas complete the meal.

Stuffed Quinoa Peppers
   Cooked quinoa, about 2 cups
   Red, green, or yellow bell peppers (1/2 to 1 per person), seeded
   Half of a sweet onion, chopped
   6-10 mushrooms, sliced
   Minced garlic
   1 package of frozen spinach (or fresh, but remember, it takes a lot)
   ½ can diced tomatoes
   Bottled salsa
   Teaspoon vinegar
   Tablespoon chili powder
   Hot chili sauce to taste
   Salt to taste

Originating in South America, the grain quinoa is high in quality protein and fiber but is gluten-free and also is low in starch. Quinoa is considered the least allergenic of all grains.

Steam the spinach until soft. At the same time, prepare the quinoa as per instructions on the box. Sauté onions, mushrooms, and seasonings in olive oil. Mix in the cooked quinoa, spinach, tomatoes, and salsa. Fill a whole or a half pepper (depending on the size of the pepper) with the mix and place in a baking dish. Sprinkle freshly grated parmesan cheese on the top and bake at 350 degrees for about 20-30 minutes. This can be a meal in itself, but also can be served with another vegetable or a salad.

Chicken/Zucchini Teriyaki
   2-4 chicken breasts cut into small pieces
   2-4 cups of zucchini squash cut into small pieces
   onion
   1-2 cups of mushrooms
   1-2 tbs. olive oil
   ½-1 cup plain or garlic hummus
   1-2 tbs. strained or plain yogurt

1-2 cups of teriyaki sauce

Cut the zucchini squash and mushrooms into small pieces. Chop up the onion. Steam the vegetables until tender. In a wok, stir-fry the chicken in olive oil. Add the steamed vegetables and mix together. Stir in the teriyaki sauce, hummus, and sour cream/plain yogurt. Heat until bubbling and serve.
Serve with steamed green beans.

Seafood Steamer
Steam unpeeled shrimp, clams, and fish or scallops seasoned with "Old Bay" or similar spices. Serve with baked red potatoes and slaw.
Slice little red potatoes in half and bake for 20 to 30 minutes with salt, pepper, a little olive oil and/or other spices on top. The potatoes can also be cooked in the lower pot of the steamer.
Slaw—any recipe will do. Here's how I make mine: Shred a bowl full of cabbage and carrots. Add enough (not too much) mayonnaise to stick it together. Add 1 to 2 tsp. of vinegar, salt, pepper, and a little mustard.

SOUPS AND CHOWDERS
Chicken vegetable stew
   2-3 boneless chicken breasts
   1-2 tbsp. olive oil
   raw mushrooms (about 2 cups, chopped)
   onion (1-2 cups)
   minced garlic
   other assorted vegetables
   vegetable or chicken broth
   1 cup uncooked brown rice
   2 tbsp. freshly minced herbs – thyme, oregano, rosemary
   salt and pepper
   1 large can crushed tomatoes
   1 can tomato puree

In a large deep stew pot, sauté 2-3 chopped up chicken breasts (free range) in 1-2 tbsp. olive oil along with the mushrooms (any kind) and the chopped onion. Add 1-2 tsp. of fresh minced garlic.

Add other vegetables to your liking. I toss in about a cup of each of the following: chopped cabbage, chopped carrots, green beans, peas, corn, a stalk of chopped celery, and 3 medium zucchinis.

Add enough water to cover all of the vegetables and several cups of organic vegetable or chicken broth for flavor. Add one cup of uncooked brown rice.

Season with 2 tbsp. of fresh minced thyme or an herb of your choice (oregano, rosemary, marjoram, and basil work well), 1 tsp. of salt, and pepper.

Bring the mixture to a boil and then reduce to a simmer for about an hour. Toward the end add the crushed tomatoes and tomato puree.

This is enough for a crowd or for several meals, and it freezes wonderfully.

Easy Vegetarian Chili
There are almost an unlimited number of chili recipes and many of them can be made without meat. The following is a recipe for a rich and healthy chili that can be made in about 10 minutes. You won't miss the meat.

  Carrots, onions, zucchini, and cabbage, chopped (2-3 cups total)
  Olive oil
  Minced garlic
  1 can of organic crushed tomatoes
  1 can of dark kidney beans, rinsed
  1 can of black beans, rinsed
  Spices include chili powder, cayenne pepper (freshly mince preferred), cumin, and salt
  Secret ingredient: 1 tablespoon of cocoa powder
  Chopped prunes and sundried tomatoes (optional)
  Mashed tempeh and/or cauliflower are excellent for thickeners

In a medium pot, sauté chopped carrots, onions, and garlic in 1 to 2 tbsp. of olive oil. Cook until the carrots are tender. Mix in one can of crushed tomatoes (look for fire roasted organic tomatoes), one can of dark red kidney beans, and one can of black beans. Add in one bay leaf, 1 to 2 tbsp. chili powder, cayenne pepper to taste, salt to taste, and 1 to 2 tsp. of cumin. Simmer for about 10 minutes.

Serve with a salad.

Moroccan Vegetable Chili

This is a very healthful dish. It is meat-free, gluten-free, and dairy-free, but the combination of flavors and spices creates a very flavorful meal.

- Vegetables--broccoli, cauliflower, carrots, onions, and red bell peppers
- Red lentils
- Macadamia nut oil (or olive oil)
- Light vinegar (such as rice wine vinegar)
- One can of diced tomatoes or tomato sauce (organic)
- Spices including: chili powder, hot chili sauce, curry paste, cumin, and salt
- Grated ginger
- Minced garlic

First prepare the red lentils. Red lentils are best if thoroughly washed until the water is clear. This usually takes four to six washings. A cup of dry lentils will absorb about 1 ½ to 2 cups of water. Bring to a boil and then simmer for about 10-15 minutes. Save the leftovers for lunch the next day.

Stir-fry or sauté about 2 cups of diced onion and peppers in 1-2 tablespoons of oil. Meanwhile, steam or microwave a handful of carrots, 1-2 sticks of broccoli and an equal amount of cauliflower.

Returning to the onions and peppers, add in the spices to your tastes. This is usually about 1-2 tablespoons of chili powder, ½ teaspoon of chili paste, a teaspoon of cumin, a tablespoon of curry paste, 1-2 teaspoons of vinegar, salt to taste, and a full teaspoon each of grated ginger and minced garlic. Stir in the lentils and the vegetables and the dish is complete. Serve alone or over brown rice.

The Best Beef Stew
   1 small sirloin steak (free-range preferred) – diced
   2 cups mushrooms – sliced in half
   1 whole onion – diced
   2 tbsp. olive oil
   4 small red potatoes - diced
   3-4 stalks of celery cut in pieces
   1 bag of peeled carrots
   1 bag frozen or fresh green beans (or green peas, corn, or butterbeans)
   1-2 tsp. garlic
   2-3 tbsp. minced herbs – rosemary, sage, & thyme
   2 tbsp. garbanzo bean flour (optional)
   2 tbsp. balsamic vinegar or red wine
   1 small can of tomato paste (organic)
   1 can diced tomatoes (organic)
   1 cup barley grain

In a stew pot sauté the steak, onions, garlic, and mushrooms in olive oil until brown. Sprinkle in the bean flour if you desire a thicker stew. Toss in everything else and cover with water. Bring to a boil and then lower to a simmer for 40-60 minutes.

Something for a Cold January Night
   1-2 large acorn squash (any winter squash)
   1-2 cups soy milk
   ½ cup cream (optional—soymilk can be substituted)
   ½ tsp. nutmeg
   ½ tsp powdered ginger
   salt and pepper to taste

Peel and half the squash. Remove the seeds. Cut into smaller pieces and boil in water until soft. Drain the water and blend the squash in a food processor. Transfer back into the pot and add soy milk, cream, and spices. Cook briefly on medium heat until bubbling.

For variation try using Garam Masala (coriander, black pepper, cumin, cardamom, and cinnamon) as the spice and add in a couple of tablespoons of coconut milk for flavor.

Serve with a fresh greens salad, gluten-free bread or crackers with thinly sliced Swiss cheese and a glass of Pinot Grigio.

Root Stew
A rich creamy stew that will make anyone like beets:
    Assorted roots such as carrots, parsnips, turnips, sweet potatoes, red potatoes, beets, leeks (or onions) – chopped into small pieces
    Several stalks of celery, chopped
    2-3 tbs fresh minced cilantro
    1-2 tsp curry powder
    1-2 tsp cumin
    ½ tsp cinnamon
    Salt and pepper
Toss all the ingredients into a large pot. Add water until the vegetables are covered. On the stove bring to a boil and then lower to a slow simmer for about one hour. The sweet potatoes will break apart and thicken the stew. To make it creamy, add a cup of soy milk just before serving.
Serve with a salad.

STANDARD AMERICAN FARE
Gingered butternut squash
This dish starts with ginger tea. Peel a piece of fresh ginger a little larger than your thumb. Slice it into thin slices and place in a tea strainer. Immerse in small pot of water and bring to a boil. When the water is barely boiling, turn off the heat and allow the tea to steep for about ten minutes. You can add in a couple of bags of regular tea if you like. Sweeten and serve hot or with ice.
Take the ginger left over from making the tea and mince finely with a knife. Mix with 1-2 tablespoons of butter and 1-2 tablespoons of brown sugar.

Split a butternut squash in half, clean out the seeds, and place with the cut side down in a baking dish with water covering the bottom. Bake at 375 until soft (30-45 minutes). Flip the squash and make several cross-ways slices into the meat of the squash with a knife. Spread the ginger mixture across the surface of the squash, pushing it down into the slices. Bake for 5-10 more minutes and serve.

Kale and beans

A large bag full of fresh kale, washed
Half an onion, chopped
Red bell pepper, chopped
Minced garlic
Minced fresh thyme and/or rosemary
One can of red beans (or any other beans)
1-2 cups of cooked rice
½ - 1 cup of vegetable broth
1-2 heaping tablespoons of apricot jam
1-2 tablespoons of balsamic vinegar
Olive oil
<1/2 teaspoon of red pepper paste or fresh-minced hot red pepper

Sauté the onion, red pepper, garlic, red pepper paste and thyme in olive oil in a large pan on medium high heat. When the onions are brown, add in the kale. Cover the pot, but open it frequently to stir. When the kale is wilted, add in the vegetable broth and all of the other ingredients. Lower the heat and simmer covered for about ten minutes. Serve.

Other greens can be used. Try it with collards or Swiss chard. This dish goes well with the gingered butternut squash.

Mashed cauliflower

Steam a head of cauliflower until soft. Chop it up in a large bowl and add in butter and soymilk. Use a food processor or hand mixer to blend until thick and smooth. Salt to taste.

Steamed vegetables

Any kind, in any combination. Try various seasonings and sauces.

Rice and beets

Okay, so I'm one of those odd individuals who liked beets from the beginning, but you can develop a taste for them and this dish will help. Peel about four fresh beets. Boil until soft. Dice into small cubes after cooling. Mix with cooked brown basmati rice, salt (to taste) and 1-2 teaspoons of balsamic vinegar.

Quinoa as a side dish

Quinoa has a texture and taste mildly reminiscent of grits. The flavor stands alone, but can be dressed up. Start with two cups of water to one cup of grain. Cook on low, covered, for about 15 minutes. Spice it up with a sauté of onions, red bell peppers, celery, garlic and fresh oregano in olive oil.

You can just use half of the quinoa for the dish and refrigerate half for breakfast. The next morning, reheat the quinoa with butter, milk (soy milk), maple syrup and raisins for a really tasty breakfast cereal.

Sweet potatoes

Wash sweet potatoes thoroughly. Stick them with a fork several times before placing in the oven. Bake them at about 375 until soft. This usually takes about 35-45 minutes.

The potatoes can also be cut into chunks and steamed or boiled until soft. Drain the water. Mash with a fork and add a little butter. At this point, you can go the usual route by adding brown sugar and cinnamon, or you can get creative: try a sprinkle of cocoa or cumin, instead.

Slaw

There are probably more different kinds of recipes for slaw than for any other single dish. It can be made in a food processor or chopped by hand. Raisins and apples add sweetness without sugar. Use a large bowl and chop enough cabbage and carrots to fill it about half full. This makes it easier to mix. The exact amount of the ingredients does not matter, but use less mayonnaise and oil than you would think necessary, just enough to coat the vegetables.

   Chopped cabbage—green, red or Savoy—or a mix of all three
   Grated carrots
   One chopped apple
   One cup raisins
   A teaspoon of mustard
   A spoonful of mayonnaise
   A dribble of canola oil
   A hint of vinegar
   Salt and pepper to taste

Mix everything together and serve. Try other variations with other spices, such as cumin and a dash of cayenne pepper.

Bahamian peas and rice

Peas and rice is a staple dish found all over the Caribbean with many derivations. Most of them contain bacon, but here is a vegetarian version. Red beans, black-eyed peas or lima beans can be used, but most commonly this dish is made with Crowder peas. There are so many variations of this recipe, that missing ingredients are never a problem.

   brown basmati rice, cooked (2-3 cups)
   Small sweet onion, diced
   2-3 stalks of celery, diced
   Olive oil.
   1 can Crowder peas, rinsed
   1 can diced organic tomatoes
   2 tablespoons of tomato paste
   2-3 tablespoons fresh minced thyme
   1-2 teaspoons minced garlic
   Small amount of hot chili paste or chopped hot pepper
   ½ -1 5.5 oz. coconut milk
   ½ cup (or less) vegetable broth
   ½ lime
   Salt to taste

In a 2-3 quart pan, sauté the onions, celery, garlic, thyme and hot pepper in a small amount of olive oil until the onions are brown. Add in all of the other ingredients and then the rice. Stir over low heat until all of the ingredients are well-mixed.

Baked fish

Any large fish such as grouper, ocean trout, or snapper will do. Place the whole fish (headed, scaled and gutted) in a large baking dish. Cut slices along the body of the fish into the flesh to allow flavors to blend. Surround the fish with sliced vegetable such as onions, celery, tomatoes, small red potatoes, red or yellow bell peppers and mushrooms. Spread minced garlic and fresh minced herbs such as oregano, thyme or rosemary on top of the fish. Dribble olive oil over the top of everything. Cover with foil. Bake at 425 for about 45 minutes, depending on the size of the fish.

Ranch beans

This recipe will make you never want to open another can of regular baked beans again.

  1 can each of white beans (cantanoli), pinto beans, and kidney beans (organic preferred), washed in a colander and drained.
  1 bell pepper, chopped (red, orange, yellow, or green)
  ½-1 sweet onion, chopped
  Minced garlic
  ¼- ½ cup of sweet BBQ sauce
  1 tablespoon chili powder
  ½ teaspoon cumin
  ½ teaspoon Mexican oregano
  Cayenne pepper to taste
  Salt to taste
  Olive oil

Sauté the peppers, onion, and garlic in olive oil until soft. Stir in all the beans and all the spices. Serve as is or bake at 350 for 15 minutes.

CASSEROLES AND BAKED DISHES

Casseroles generally require more prep and kitchen time, but the tradeoff is being able to store them in the refrigerator or freezer. I never make just one lasagna—there are always two, one for dinner and one for the freezer. Casseroles are perfect to serve a crowd.

As with other dishes, do not worry about specific ingredients or the amounts of ingredients. Feel free to add or subtract items according to your particular tastes. That is what cooking is all about.

Grouper Moussaka

This is a light and healthy version of what is traditionally a heavy meat dish. Grouper is used here because it is a less oily white meat fish with few bones and it soaks up all the flavors of the Moussaka. Other fish such as flounder or halibut work just fine, too. This recipe can also be made vegetarian by omitting the fish and substituting tempeh.

1-2 lbs. of fresh grouper, preferably in one filet
1 large or 2 medium eggplants
1 medium sweet onion, sliced and chopped
1 package of fresh mushrooms, sliced
3 medium tomatoes (sliced into small chunks) or one can crushed tomatoes
1 yellow or red bell pepper
1 6oz. can of tomato paste
1 handful of fresh basil, oregano, and a little rosemary, minced
1 teaspoon cinnamon
½ teaspoon tumeric
Lots of minced garlic
Shredded parmesan cheese
2-3 tablespoons olive oil
Salt to taste

Béchamel sauce

2-3 tablespoons olive oil

4 tablespoons of garbanzo bean flour (Found in most health food stores, this is a tasty flour substitute. Hummus can be used if this is not available.)
2 cups of soy milk
½ cup shredded parmesan cheese
Dash or two of nutmeg

Peel and slice the eggplant into ½ inch thick slices. Lightly salt the pieces and lay them into a colander for about 20 minutes. Everyone says this is to allow the bitter juices to sweat out, but I have never noticed much difference when I cook eggplant without this step. Place the eggplant on a baking sheet and bake for about 20 minutes in an oven pre-heated to 375.

While waiting on the eggplant, prepare the Béchamel sauce. In a saucepan, whisk the garbanzo bean flower and olive oil together on medium heat until bubbly. I sometimes add a teaspoon of butter. Set aside to cool completely. Add the soy milk and slowly reheat, stirring constantly. Continue until thickened. Stir in the cheese and nutmeg, and set aside.

Sauté the mushrooms, onions, and peppers in olive oil until tender. Add in the tomatoes, tomato paste, garlic, herbs, and spices. Simmer for about 10-15 minutes.

Place the fish in the middle of a large baking dish. Slice the eggplant into smaller sections and layer around the fish. Layer the mushroom mixture over the top of the fish and eggplant. Pour the béchamel sauce across the top. Bake covered with foil for about 35-45 minutes. During the last 10 minutes remove the foil and sprinkle parmesan cheese over the top. Serve with a lettuce salad.

Wild rice and turkey

2 cups of cooked brown rice
2 cups of cooked wild rice
2-3 cups baked turkey or chicken, chopped into small chunks
1-2 tbsp. of garbanzo bean flour or unbleached flour
2 tbsp. olive oil or macadamia nut oil
Chopped celery, onion and mushrooms

1 cup soymilk
1 cup vegetable or chicken broth
broccoli, several stalks chopped into small pieces
1 egg
lemon
1-2 tbsp. mayonnaise or hummus
salt and pepper
fresh rosemary, minced.

In a saucepan, sauté 1 to 2 tbsp. of garbanzo bean flour in a couple of tbsp. of olive oil. Cook about one minute, cool, and then stir in one cup of soy milk and one cup of chicken or vegetable broth. Cook on medium heat, stirring continuously, until thickened.

Meanwhile, lightly steam or microwave the broccoli and sauté the onions, celery and mushrooms in oil.

Lightly beat one egg yolk with a little fresh lemon. Slowly mix in a spoonful of the broth/soymilk mixture and then pour it all back into the saucepan. Add in 1 to 2 tbsp. of either mayonnaise or hummus and heat through.

Mix this sauce with the turkey, broccoli, vegetables, brown rice and wild rice. Salt and pepper to taste. Rosemary is also a nice spice for this dish.

Transfer to a casserole dish. Grate fresh parmesan cheese on top. Bake at 350 for 20 to 30 minutes, or until brown.

Prepare more than one dish at a time and freeze the extras for later use.

Vegetable Lasagna
½ box whole wheat lasagna noodles
1 eggplant
Several cups of vegetables—zucchini, onions, mushrooms, spinach, broccoli, carrots (any combination)
1 tsp minced garlic
1 tbs minced fresh oregano
1 tsp fresh minced basil

1 jar pasta sauce

Filling
　½ cup low fat cottage cheese
　½ cup low fat ricotta cheese
　1 egg
　½ cup mozzarella cheese (optional)
　½ cup parmesan cheese

Slice eggplant into ½ inch slices and place in a colander to allow the slices to "sweat." Pat dry with a paper towel. This removes some of the bitterness. Lay the eggplant on a cooking sheet seasoned with cooking spray. Bake at 350ºF for about 15 minutes, or until lightly browned. Boil the noodles until tender and drain. (Add about one tsp of olive oil to the water to prevent the noodles from sticking together.) At the same time, steam or microwave (6 minutes on high) all of the vegetables, basil, oregano, and garlic until tender. In a separate bowl, mix the cottage cheese, ricotta, cheese, egg, mozzarella cheese, and parmesan cheese.

For the layering process use a deep baking dish roughly 9 x 11. Most commonly three layers of noodles are used, but this recipe can be made lighter with less filling and two layers of sparsely spaced noodles. Also less mozzarella and ricotta cheese can be used. Layering goes like this: Start with a layer of noodles on the bottom. Add a layer of eggplant slices (or ½ eggplant and ½ browned ground beef). Thinly spread eggplant with the cheese mixture. Drizzle with some of the sauce. Add another layer of noodles. A layer of vegetables comes next. More sauce goes on top of the vegetables. Top with a final layer of sauce. Sprinkle with mozzarella and parmesan cheese. Cover with foil and place in the oven at 350º for 30 min. Remove the foil during the last 15 minutes to allow the cheese to brown.

This dish can be prepared and then kept in the refrigerator for several days or frozen prior to baking. Make two lasagnas and freeze one for later use.

Sweet Potato Burritos
   4 cups sweet potatoes, cooked and mashed
   Can of black beans, rinsed and drained
   Can of kidney beans, rinsed and drained
   1 onion, chopped
   1 T. minced garlic
   3 T. soy sauce
   3-4 tsp. prepared mustard
   1-2 T. chili powder
   2 tsp. ground cumin
   Just a dash of cayenne pepper
   Whole wheat tortillas
   Shredded cheese (optional)
   Salsa (optional)

Sauté onions and garlic in 1-2 tbsp. of olive oil. In a large bowl, mash beans slightly and mix with the spices, onion and garlic. Add a bit of water if stiff. Mix in the mashed sweet potatoes.

Spoon mixture into tortillas, fold, and place in casserole dish. Spread salsa on top. Bake at for about 15-20 minutes.

These freeze quite well. Wrap them separately and place into a freezer box for quick meals.

Sweet and Sour Winter Roasted Vegetables
The aromas in the kitchen and the warmth of the oven while this dish is cooking are enough to melt away any cold winter night.
   Beets
   Carrots
   Brussels sprouts
   Mushrooms
   Leeks or red onions
   Sweet potatoes
   Cauliflower
   Prunes (secret ingredient)

Olive oil—about ¼ cup
Maple syrup—about ¼ cup
Apple cider vinegar—about ¼ cup
Ground sage
Fresh or dry minced thyme
Salt and pepper

Cut vegetables into chunks—enough to fill a 2 quart container. Steam the vegetables for about five minutes. Place them into a large baking dish and drizzle olive oil across the vegetables. Sprinkle sage, thyme, salt and pepper across all of the vegetables. Bake at 400 degrees for 20 minutes, covered. Mix the vinegar and maple syrup well and pour over the mixture. Bake for another 20 minutes. Take off the cover for part of the time to allow the vegetables to brown slightly.

For many more recipes and extended guidelines to healthy eating, log onto <u>www.vitalplan.com</u>.

Acknowledgements

First and foremost, I would like to thank my patients for all they have taught me over the years.

I would like to thank my wife, Meg, for her exceptional editing talents, without which, the book would have been impossible. Her professional insights and input have been invaluable. Having someone close at hand with training in science has helped me stay on the straight and narrow.

I would like to thank my daughter, Braden, for her exceptional organizational skills in bringing this edition to print once again.

Leslie McCombs-Porter again deserves my thanks for editing the first edition.

Dawn Brock, who has an eye for detail and originality, formatted the original book into readable form.

Thanks to Amy Ballard for her efforts in formatting the new edition.

My thanks to staff members present at my office during the time the book was written. Each of them contributed in positive ways. A special thanks to Christie Fulcher, R.N., who also helped proofread on several occasions and provided input and feedback on a daily basis while the health program was being created.

REFERENCES

Some writing is the result of specific research with the primary purpose of conveying information. This type of writing is essential in a book of this sort and should be backed by specific references. The primary references cited were used to research factual information.

Secondary references provided factual information as well as opinions or theories worth considering. Some information, such as the theories about alkalinity and osteoporosis, is less absolute but helps guide the reader toward a specific goal and provides food for thought.

Much of the writing in the book happened spontaneously—often as a result of searching for better ways to explain concepts to patients. During the time I was immersed in writing the book, ideas would often come while on a long walk or in the shower and would end up scribbled on snips of paper, later to be included. This type of writing generally does not result from well-defined references, but is the consequence of years of accumulated knowledge, synthesized through common sense into a workable form.

In many places in the book, reference is made to specific web sites or specific books and authors. These resources are listed here in hopes that readers will use them to pursue greater knowledge.

Primary references

Harper's Biochemistry, 25th Edition, A Large Medical Book
    Robert K. Murray, M.D., PhD., Daryl K. Granner, M.D.
    Peter D. Mayes, PhD., DSC, Victor W. Rodwell, PhD.
    McGraw-Hill, Copyright 2000, 1996, 1993, 1990, 1988
    ISBN 0-8385-3684-0

Review of Medical Physiology, 20th Edition
    William F. Ganong, M.D.
    Lange Medical Books, McGraw-Hill 1999
    ISBN 0-8385-8282-6

Advanced Nutrition and Human Metabolism, 3rd Edition
    James L. Groff, Sareen S. Gropper
    Wadsworth, Copyright 2000
    ISBN 0-534-55521-7

Textbook of Functional Medicine
    David S. Jones, M.D., Editor in Chief
    Institute for Functional Medicine
    Copyright 2005
    ISBN 0-9773713-0-1

Modern Nutrition Health and Disease, 9th Edition
    Editor Donna Bulado
    Williams and Wilkins
    Copyright 1999
    ISBN 0-683-30769-X

The Relaxation and Stress Reduction Workbook, 5th Edition
    Martha Davis, PhD.
    Elizabeth Robbins Eshelman, MSW
    Matthew McKay, PhD.
    New Harbinger Publications, Inc.
    Copyright 2000
    ISBN 1-57224-214-0

Modern Concepts in Biochemistry, 3rd Edition
    Robert C. Bohinski
    Allyn and Bacon, Inc.
    Copyright 1979
    ISBN 0-205-06541-X

The Relaxation Response
    Herbert Benson, M.D.
    Avon Books, Inc.
    Copyright 1975
    ISBN 0-380-81595-8

Meditation for Dummies
    Stephan Bodian
    Wiley Publishing Company, Inc., Indianapolis, Indiana
    Copyright 1999

The Open Focus Brain
    Les Fehmi, PhD., Jim Robbins
    Trumpeter Books
    Copyright 2007
    ISBN 987-I-590301-376-4

Drawing on the Ride Side of the Brain
    Betty Edwards
    G. P. Putnam's Sons
    Copyright 1987
    ISBN 0-87477-513-2

The Healthiest Diet in the World
    Nikki and David Goldbeck
    Penguin Putnam, Inc., Dutton Books
    Copyright 1998
    ISBN 0-525-94282-3

Estrogen Metabolism and the Diet-Cancer Connection: Rational for Assessing the Ratio of Urinary Hydroxylated Estrogen Metabolites
    Richard S. Lord, PhD, Bradley Bongiovanni, ND, and J. Alexander Bralley, PhD, CCN.
    Alternative Medicine Review, Volume 7, Number 2, 2002

Foods to Fight Cancer, Essential foods to help prevent cancer
    Richard Beliveau, Ph.D. and Denis Gingras, Ph.D.
    DK Publishing, New York, New York
    Copyright 2007
    ISBN 978-0-7566-2867-3

Detoxify or Die
    Sherry A. Rogers, M.D
    Sand Key Company, Inc.
    Copyright 2002
    ISBN: 1-887202-04-8

Breaking the Vicious Cycle
    Elaine Gottschall, B.A., M.Sc.
    The Kirkton Press, Baltimore, Maryland
    Copyright 2004
    ISBN 0-9692768-1-8

Biofeedback, A Practitioner's Guide, 3rd edition
    Mark S. Schwartz and Frank Andrasik, editors
    The Guilford Press, New York, New York
    Copyright 2003
    ISBN-13: 978-1-57230-845-9

Laboratory Evaluations in Molecular Medicine
    J Alexander Bralley, PhD, CCN and Richard S. Lord, PhD
    The Institute for Advances in Molecular Medicine, Norcross, Ga.
    Copyright 2001
    ISBN-10: 0-9673949-1-0

Secondary references

Healing with Whole Foods, Asian Traditions and Modern Nutrition, 3rd Edition
    Paul Pitchford
    North Atlantic Books, Berkeley, California
    Copyright 1993
    ISBN 1-55643-430-8

Staying Healthy with Nutrition
    Elson M. Haas, M.D.
    Copyright 1992
    Celestial Arts, Berkeley, California
    ISBN 0-89087-481-6

Overcoming Thyroid Disorders, 2nd edition
    David Brownstein, M.D.
    Medical Alternatives Press
    Copyright 2008
    ISBN 978-0-960882-2-9

Foods That Fight Pain
    Neal Barnard, M.D.
    Three Rivers Press   New York, New York
    Copyright 1998
    ISBN 0-609-80436-7

The Natural Testosterone Plan, for sexual health and energy
    Stephen Harrod Buhner
    Healing Arts Press   Rochester, Vermont
    Copyright 2007
    ISBN 978-1-59477-168-2

The Lyme Disease Solution
    Kenneth B. Singleton, M.D., M.P.H.
    Brown Books, Dallas, Texas
    Copyright 2008
    ISBN-13: 978-1-934812-00-6

Cruising World
    October 2008 "Skimming the Sands of Sable"

National Geographic
    November 2005 "The Secrets of Living Longer"

Diet, Life Expectancy, and Chronic Disease—Studies of Seventh Day Adventists and Other Vegetarians (reference for the Heidelberg Vegetarian Study)
Gary Fraser
Oxford Press
Copyright 2003

Additional references for the new edition

The Okinawa Program
Bradley J. Willcox, M.D., Craig Willcox, Ph.D., and Makoto Suzuki, M.D.
Three Rivers Press, New York
Copyright 2001
ISBN 0-609-80750-1
(This source was read after completion of the book, but is important because it supports all concepts discussed in the book with a population study.)

Wheat Belly
William Davis, MD
Rondale, Inc.
Copyright 2011
ISBN 978-1-60961-154-5
(Though this reference did not become available until the end of the rewrite, it became an invaluable reference for confirming suspicions about wheat and is an excellent source of information. This reference is highly recommended for individuals suffering from wheat sensitivity.)

Website references
Toxins:
www.pollutioninpeople.org
www.chemicalbodyburden.org
www.ourstolenfuture.org

Gastrointestinal disorders:
www.breakingtheviciouscycle.info

Alkaline water:
www.hightechhealth.com

FIR sauna:
www.hightechhealth.com

Healthy food:
www.barleyfoods.org *recipes using barley grain*
www.quinoa.net *recipes using quinoa*
www.sunnylandfarms.com *resource for fresh nuts*
www.eatwild.com *resource for finding local free-range meat*
www.oceansalive.org *resource for finding healthy seafood*
www.organicconsumer.org *resource for finding organic food*
www.whfoods.com *extensive resource for information about food*
www.localharvest.org *resource for finding locally harvested foods*
www.bobsredmill.com *resource for organic grain products*

Healthy products:
www.realgoods.com *resource for many environmentally favorable products*
www.seventhgeneration.com *"green" household products*

Relaxation:
www.TheRelaxationCompany.com *source for Dr. Jeffrey Thompson's CD's*
www.openfocus.com

Nutritional supplements:
www.naturaldatabase.com *paid source for scientific data about nutraceuticals*
www.naturalstandard.com *paid source of scientific data about nutraceuticals*
www. vitalplan.com *source of premium natural supplements*

REVITALIZE™ YOUR LIFE
Join hundreds of others who are enjoying optimal health by living the VITAL PLAN™

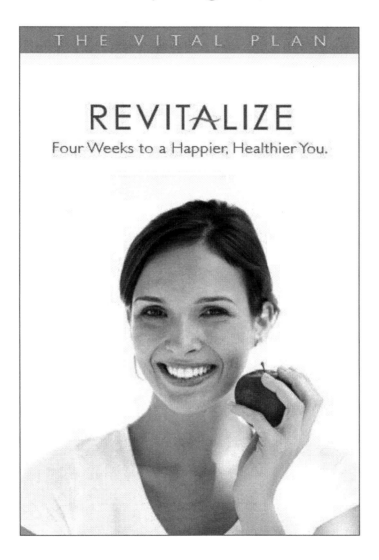

The 4 week REVTIALIZE Optimal Wellness Guide is available at <u>www.vitalplan.com</u>

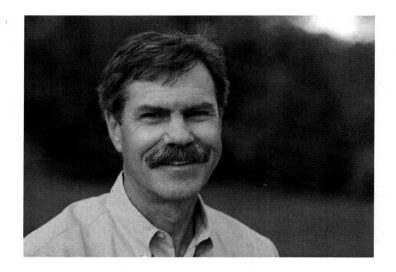

Dr. Rawls attended medical school at Bowman Gray School of Medicine (Wake Forest University). He is board certified in obstetrics and gynecology and maintains a medical license in the state of North Carolina. He also has extensive training in what is defined as alternative medicine and has undergone certification training in holistic medicine. This training is complemented by a passion for the study of concepts in natural healing.

Dr. Rawls resides on the coast in North Carolina, where his other passions include sailing and kitesurfing. He lives with his wife of thirty years, who teaches biology at the local community college. Together they live and promote concepts of wellness. His daughter, a passionate entrepreneur, oversees development of Vital Plan, Inc. His son is presently enrolled in medical school in Charleston, SC.